Praise for

OF MY OWN MAKING

"*Of My Own Making* is a beautifully written book that takes you on a journey of growth through the deep-rooted traumas of our pasts. Part memoir, part manual, Daria has offered readers a chance to reflect and release alongside her own brilliant story. A must-read for those ready to face the past and move forward with compassion, hope, and optimism."

—Rachel Cargle, author of *A Renaissance of Our Own*

"Burke writes with a captivating honesty and endless curiosity. *Of My Own Making* is a timely reminder that no matter where we are in life, the past manages to find its way in. It's how we handle it that shapes who we really are."

—Ellen Vora, MD, psychiatrist and
author of *The Anatomy of Anxiety*

"This is a story of hope, resilience, and the indomitable spirit of a woman who defied the odds to carve out her own path. With masterful prose that is both poetic and incisive, she invites readers into her world, exploring the intersections of education, career, and identity. Each page reveals her profound insights into the human condition, as she navigates the shadows of her past and their impact on her present. As she uncovers her story, you'll find yourself rooting for her triumphs and celebrating her unwavering spirit."

—David Ambroz, author of *A Place Called Home*

DARIA BURKE

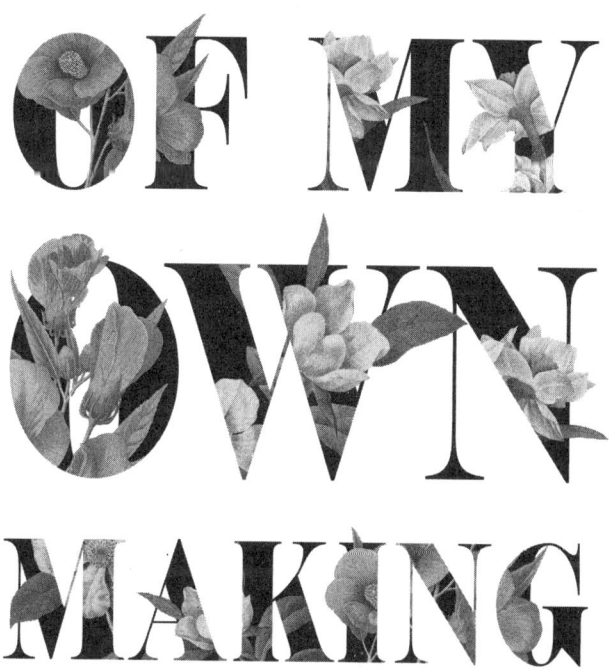

OF MY OWN MAKING

A MEMOIR

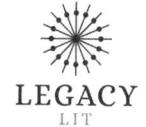

LEGACY
LIT

New York Boston

Copyright © 2025 by Daria Burke

Cover design by Peter Garceau. Cover images by Getty images.

Cover copyright © 2025 by Hachette Book Group, Inc.

Legacy Lit

Hachette Book Group

1290 Avenue of the Americas

New York, NY 10104

LegacyLitBooks.com

@LegacyLitBooks

First Edition: April 2025

Legacy Lit is an imprint of Grand Central Publishing. The Legacy Lit name and logo are registered trademarks of Hachette Book Group, Inc.

The publisher is not responsible for websites (or their content) that are not owned by the publisher.

The Hachette Speakers Bureau provides a wide range of authors for speaking events. To find out more, go to hachettespeakersbureau.com or email HachetteSpeakers@hbgusa.com.

Legacy Lit books may be purchased in bulk for business, educational, or promotional use. For information, please contact your local bookseller or the Hachette Book Group Special Markets Department at special.markets@hbgusa.com.

Print book interior design by Jeff Stiefel

Library of Congress Cataloging-in-Publication Data

Names: Burke, Daria, author.

Title: Of my own making : a memoir / Daria Burke.

Description: First edition. | New York : Legacy Lit, 2025.

Identifiers: LCCN 2024047461 | ISBN 9781538766804 (hardcover) | ISBN 9781538766828 (ebook)

Subjects: LCSH: Burke, Daria. | Adult child abuse victims—Biography. | Motivational speakers—United States—Biography. | African American women executives—Biography. | Psychic trauma in children. | Resilience (Personality trait) | Rehabilitation.

Classification: LCC RC569.5.C55 B86 2025 | DDC 362.76/4092—dc23/eng/20250122

LC record available at https://lccn.loc.gov/2024047461

ISBNs: 978-1-5387-6680-4 (hardcover), 978-1-5387-6682-8 (ebook)

Printed in the United States of America

LSC-C

Printing 1, 2025

For the little girl
who dreamed of my becoming,
and for all the versions
who helped me get here.

CONTENTS

CONTENTS

OF MY OWN MAKING

PROLOGUE

On my thirty-fifth birthday, I stood at the threshold of a gate that opened to the quiet grandeur of a private estate in East Hampton, a sanctuary enveloped by a hundred-acre preserve that spoke of exclusivity and retreat. This wasn't just a seven-bedroom house nestled in the woods of Wainscott; it was a tribute to my journey from meager beginnings to stand, humbled yet proud, at the doorstep of a home (albeit rented for the weekend) that promised solace and celebration, a pause to honor the journey that had led me here, from a past that was far less forgiving. It was here that I decided to mark the passage of another year, surrounded by my closest friends, souls who had walked many of those miles beside me.

There is nothing like early October in the Hamptons. After the summer crowds have long dissipated but before the thick rustle of leaves, when the weather remains warm enough to enjoy outdoor dining and walks to the beach. But this weekend, there was a torrential rainstorm that would ask us instead to languish in the comfort of deep, plush sofas and each other's company. In the quiet solitude before their arrival, I placed a small welcome gift and note upon each bed and imagined their faces as they would enter the grounds past the manicured ballet of hedges and a fountain that seemed to dance straight out of a Fitzgerald dream.

The next evening, we gathered at the long dining table overlooking the pool as the private chef I'd hired served tuna tartare in martini glasses, followed by three more courses and several bottles of wine and champagne. Dessert was my favorite—banana pudding from Magnolia Bakery. In that moment, wrapped in the perfect harmony of friends and fortune, I celebrated not just a birthday but a triumph—the ascent to the pinnacle of beauty, an executive among the corporate elite, encircled by a family of my own choosing.

After dinner, we moved to the living room and settled in to spar with humor and darkness with Cards Against Humanity. Yet, amid the revelry, a lighthearted query from a friend—"Who wants to smoke?"—severed the night in two. Half of the group headed outside to light a joint.

Not this. Not here.

I couldn't make it stop. Any of it. It was escalating too fast.

I hurried myself to the kitchen, unable to make sense of what I was experiencing as tears streamed down my face.

My chest tightened as though a vise gripped my lungs. I was no longer in the Hamptons celebrating my birthday. Suddenly I had fallen into a silo of the past, snatched through a doorway where the once-was becomes what is happening now. There, I am in Detroit again, small and quiet, my mother and her friends smoking crack in the basement of my childhood home.

"Are you okay?" The concern in Nicky's voice pulled me back, her hand reaching out to me, as if she could pull me back across the years.

Logically, I knew where I was, but I couldn't breathe, and I couldn't stop crying.

"Yes," I started to lie, retreating into myself. But I couldn't lie to Nicky given everything she knew.

"No, I'm not okay," I admitted, my voice a broken murmur. "She knows about my family and how I feel about drugs. How could she possibly have thought that this was okay?"

Nicky, ever understanding, suggested in the way that a mediating middle child would, "Maybe she didn't realize..."

"Yeah. I guess," I managed, the words as weak as a baby's first steps.

I collected myself enough to poke my head into the living room, telling everyone that I'd had too much to drink and was turning in for the night. Finally upstairs and alone, I curled into the fetal position and rocked myself to sleep, rationalizing that I was just weepy from all the wine.

There are some things that hurt so much that we don't want to remember, a compelling enough reason to try to forget. Some sorrows so deep that they require more than mere words or time to heal. They linger in the margin, waiting to be acknowledged and understood.

PART

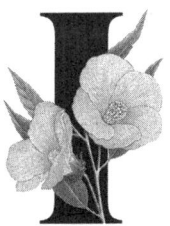

ROOTS

The blood of your parents is not lost in you.

—Menelaus, the *Odyssey*

1

GRIEF & GHOSTS

I measure every Grief I meet
With narrow, probing, Eyes;
I wonder if It weighs like Mine,
Or has an Easier size.

—Emily Dickinson, Poem 561

I f my mother's grief was to be loud, mine had to be
silent.

Mama could wail and yell and curse, her sorrow unraveling in front of us like a story too painful to tell but too heavy to hold. Her cries could crash against the walls, reverberate through the house, and settle into the corners like dust. There was no escaping her grief; it stretched across every room, swallowing all the air.

I never knew which mother I would wake up to. Some mornings she was brittle, holding herself together just enough to make breakfast. Other days, she was a storm, her emotions swirled and thrashed, unpredictable and violent. I learned to become whoever I needed to be to get through the moment, to shape myself around her mood, like water taking the form of whatever container it found itself in. With the agility of an acrobat, I tiptoed around the edges of her wild swings, navigating the minefield of her emotions. It was an act of self-preservation, this silence, an unsentimental recognition of the hierarchy of pain that governed our lives. My grand-mother's passing was my mother's agony. It was her mother who had departed, her history of love, her heartache and her loss laid bare for the world to witness. And I knew, in the way children somehow know, that there was no room for both of us in that grief. So I buried mine, deep, where it wouldn't be seen, where it wouldn't make noise, because there wasn't enough room for two hearts to break in the same house.

I was only seven, but Grandma was also mine. Our bond didn't need words, didn't need to be defined to be deeply felt. She was my person. Her lap was my sanctuary, her laughter, bright and full, was my lullaby. She helped shape my world, and bridged the gaps my mother could not. My parents had married young, kids playing house before they knew what it really meant. Their brief union culminated in two daughters—me, then Leah fourteen months later—before its dissolution when I was two years old. I don't remember my father being there and I don't remember him leaving. Mama never sounded happy when she talked about him, even the early times. So, I learned early: Don't ask, don't tell. To this day, I only know a vague story of them meeting through one of my aunts who was my mother's classmate, but not what brought them together.

But Grandma was always there. Her love was an unspoken vow, a commitment to be the pillar of our little quartet. She assumed the role of co-parent and the steady force that I believe held our lives together, a fact that did not register as odd back then. I was too young to know that I was supposed to have a mom and dad at home. My world was the way it was.

Grandma was a constant presence in a world that was undoubtedly crumbling. She visited us daily, a ritual more stoic than sentimental, after the demands of her own day's responsibilities. In her, my mother, a mere twenty-three and already marked by the obligations of two toddler daughters, found not only a guiding force but a partner in navigating the storm of early adulthood and the uncharted territory of single parenthood. My mother stayed home even after we were school age, which also meant that she didn't work. Grandma was the silent force that defied the odds stacked against us.

I remember her love not in the words she spoke, but in the comfort her stillness offered. The way she'd let me curl up beside her in bed or the way she'd let me half drape myself over her lap as she read on the sofa, little arms on bigger ones. As I drifted toward sleep, I'd open my eyes and remember to share something "hilarious" from school, always met with her gentle smile. That smile—the one that said she was listening, that she cared—was all I needed to know I was safe, secure, and loved.

Her presence was singular. Her absence loomed larger than life itself. The last time I saw Grandma, she looked serene in a mint-green dress, her body laid to rest in a pearlescent coffin. The woman who had once been so full of life, whose hands had tended to me daily with unyielding love, now lay still, her fingers crossed delicately over her belly as if she were holding the last of her own breath. I had never been to a funeral before. I had only the hints of a child's understanding of death, but the pain was profound. She had been snatched away in a moment so violent, so final, that even now, it claws at my insides.

My uncle Frank and my cousin, Nikki, had initially chosen a different dress for the burial—a brand-new A-line sheath, white with pink roses. Something pretty. But they were told that the neckline was too low to conceal the injuries on her chest and neck, so they chose the green dress from her closet. On November 14, 1987, we said goodbye to Grandma, and though she'd been the heartbeat of our family, I stood dry-eyed as we lowered her into the ground. I was seven and she was gone before I knew how to feel. I balled up my grief and stashed it away, like a box of tangled Christmas lights too overwhelming to sort through and put away neatly for later use.

My mother went to war with grief and lost. Whereas

I remember her as free-spirited and outgoing, in the wake of Grandma's death she became a stranger to me, running from or perhaps chasing demons that only she could see. We would sing and dance in the living room to her favorite music and I would stay up well past a child's bedtime to perform my best pantomime to Teena Marie's "Out on a Limb" for her friends when I was barely school age. It was as if a curtain fell, hiding her from herself and the world. She often spoke out of necessity, to summon us to eat or clean something we'd left out of place. Lost in a private anguish, the mother I had known disappeared, and I grew up a silent witness to her unraveling. Addiction pulled her quickly into its grasp, and I watched, terrified, as a crack- and cocaine-fueled storm took residence in her, one that raged and howled, leaving me to seek shelter within myself.

I became adept at fading into the background, a shadow that observed her descent from the safest possible distance. It had been neither a deliberate nor a conscious decision, to enter into this unspoken contract with the universe—to become the stable, unflinching observer, even if it meant suppressing my own needs. This emotional exit strategy was a trick designed to shield me from the pain of it all. A child's mind, unable to process the emotional violence of trauma, retreats into a self-protective cocoon of detachment. This was easy enough to do; there was no adult guiding me through the process of putting my feelings into words. No new routines to replace Grandma's daily visits or discussion of how we would live without her. No rituals to honor her memory. Maybe they couldn't. Maybe they were too consumed by their own loss. Maybe they thought I was too young to understand, too young to feel the full brunt of what had happened. But I felt it. I just didn't have the words for it. Thirty years later, the tears came.

On a mundane Wednesday evening in 2017, one like countless others, I left work later than planned. A car service sat waiting for me outside the Facebook offices on Park Avenue, where I led one of the company's largest portfolios of beauty and fashion retail advertising clients in North America. As I opened the door, I asked the driver if he wouldn't mind taking Park Avenue uptown and then through the park to my building on the Upper West Side. I had lived in New York City for more than a decade at this point, and my apartment was just a block from Central Park. But for all its orchestrated wildness, the park was still a balm to me, a respite from the urgency and ambition of the city. After a long day at the office, it calmed me to see so many trees, their lushness and greenery balancing out the hard lines and harder pace of the city. They were reminders that a world existed beyond the hustle and the deadlines, beyond the incessant need to be somewhere, to be someone.

As I sank into the back seat, I scrolled through my phone, contemplating dinner. I landed on my favorite ground beef tacos from the Great Burrito on the Upper West Side. They could be delivered in about twenty minutes, and I had gotten quite good at timing the delivery of my order for about seven minutes after I made it home. In seven minutes, I could exchange pleasantries with the doorman, check the mail, ride the elevator up to my sixth-floor apartment, wash my hands, and change clothes for the evening. Dinner arrived and I plated my tacos with extra guac, poured a can of Perrier Lime over ice, and settled onto the sofa to eat and watch TV before bed. Three-quarters into whatever I was watching, something suddenly made me think of my grandmother, compelling me to grab my laptop and search her name.

I was hoping to find her obituary, and I vaguely recalled my mother mentioning that the *Detroit Free Press* had written about her death, but my initial search came up empty. I decided to shift my focus to the newspaper's archive page, wondering what I might find among the more than three million pages and clippings dating as far back as 1837. There, I searched my grandmother's name, this time with success, as a single thumbnail appeared, followed by a headline: "Freeway crash kills Detroit woman." Heart pounding, I switched the TV off. It was the November 8, 1987, report of the car accident that had claimed my grandmother's life. My hands shook as I signed up for a free trial to access the article, overriding the paywall that stood between me and my history.

As I scrolled down the page, a photograph came into view, pinning me back against the sofa. My eyes locked on the horrific black-and-white image, one that would be forever burned into my consciousness. In the photo's background, two police officers stand on the highway shoulder huddling over a piece of paper, while another one stands facing the verge, observing the onlookers up on the street level. Two more officers stand in the foreground—one scribbling notes, the other staring intently as together they survey the wreckage.

Finally forcing myself to look toward the center of the frame, I focused on the haunting remains of my grandmother's car. The roof of her navy hatchback is peeled back like paint on an old house, the entire back half of the car having collapsed into itself, as if it bore the weight of all that was lost that day. The car's left rear tire had plunged into the back of the driver's seat, its impact molding the seat into a deformed arch around it. The speed of force had pushed the seat cushion all the way under the dashboard, leaving no room for a human body. The steering wheel hangs above the crumpled seat. The only remaining door, on the driver's side, is open. The keys are still in the ignition as if awaiting her return.

My breath hitched, heart thundering against ribs that suddenly felt too small. Time fractured, split into a before and an after with the sharpness of the broken glass in the picture. A cry escaped my lips, then morphed into a primal scream that came from a place untouched by time. Though I had known about the details of the crash for years, seeing that photo, I wailed like I had just gotten the news, like I hadn't known about the accident my entire life, like I had been there to watch as she was hurtled through the front windshield. Uncontrollable sobs shook my body, as I felt pulled into my younger self. I wept for my grandmother, and I wept for myself—for the thirty years I had not been able to cry. The tears came from a place so deep within me, I felt like I wouldn't survive them. I sat on my sofa, held in a liminal space, suspended between past and present.

I took a sip of the sparkling water, which burned my tender throat. Through tears I read the brief report:

> State troopers examine the remains of a 1983 Ford Escort, whose driver, Effie Mae Bogard, 55, of Detroit, was killed Sunday when her car stalled or ran out of gas in the center eastbound lane of I-96 near Livernois in Detroit about 11:15 a.m. and was rammed from behind by another vehicle. No one else was injured in the crash, which closed a portion of the freeway for two hours. State police said the car immediately behind the Escort swerved out of the way when the Escort stopped, but that the next car in the lane could not stop in time. The impact pushed a rear wheel of the Escort into the passenger compartment. Bogard was dead on arrival at Henry Ford Hospital. State police said that the accident was under investigation, and

that the driver who hit Bogard's car was not
held or charged.

What they didn't know was that Grandma was not one
to run out of gas. Whenever her car reached half a tank, she
would immediately refill it. That Grandma had driven past
the freeway exit to our house and was only seven minutes
away from her church. That we had been waiting for her to
pick us up that morning and that she always kept her word.
That this was never supposed to happen to her. When she
wasn't working or visiting with my mother, my sister, and me
at our house, Grandma was at Carter Metropolitan Chris-
tian Methodist Episcopal Church, leading a committee
meeting, attending a Bible study, or helping prepare for the
next wedding or funeral. She was often one of the first people to volunteer to bring homemade chicken and dumplings
to an ailing or grieving parishioner, folks the pastor called
"the sick and shut in."

Faithful church attendance with Grandma was central
to our family routine. It followed, then, that the entire congregation knew Effie's daughter, Carolyn—my mother—and
her two identically-dressed girls. I'd grown accustomed to
the exuberant chirping of "They're so cute!" and the double
take—"Are they twins?" directed at my mother, while their
eyes remained fixed on us. "No. They're fourteen months
apart. To the day," she'd say each time. Ever the performer,
she adored the attention, granting hugs and handshakes to

fellow parishioners before an usher, or my grandmother, escorted us to a pew toward the front of the church.

Sunday, November 8, 1987, had mirrored many Sundays in our preparations for church. We climbed out of our beds as my mother entered our room singing, "Riiiise and shiiiine." She poured us each a bowl of cereal, a light breakfast meant to tide us over through Sunday service. Mama always took great care in getting us ready for church: our hair, not one strand out of place; matching dresses usually gifted by my grandmother; and patent leather Mary Janes that she paired with tights in winter and ruffled socks in summer. Then she would spend another half hour or so getting herself dressed. Naturally stunning, my mother didn't wear much makeup. Her routine was minimal—two swipes of berry-colored lipstick and a touch of mascara after removing her curlers, putting on gold hoop earrings, and stepping into her pantyhose. She always wore pantyhose to church. I would watch her roll each side down to little disks, sliding them over one foot and then the other before drawing them up her long legs and over her lean, soft curves, a ritual that captivated me.

Leah and I were allowed to sit and watch cartoons while we waited for Grandma to arrive. I don't remember how long we waited. When you're a kid, time moves so slowly that you never know how long anything is supposed to take. I do remember the worry that invaded my mother's face as we waited patiently, and then less patiently, as our thick tights and crinoline ruffles began to stifle and scratch. We waited a while longer and eventually, the phone rang. It was someone from Henry Ford Hospital asking if my mother was the daughter of an Effie Bogard. In fact, she was her only daughter, and at twenty-eight, the youngest of my grandmother's four children. The person on the phone said that Grandma had been in a car accident and that we should come to the hospital right away.

There was no goodbye.

I stood up from the sofa, my body heavy and dull, as if emerging from a trance. A dam had broken inside me. Something had been stirred, summoned by an unseen force. By the remnants of that fateful day, captured in monochrome stillness. My grief, which had been in a deep freeze, was thawing, and suddenly, I was confronting the untamed and unnamed emotions imprisoned in me all those years.

With swollen eyes, I looked around my apartment. There were the polished hardwood floors, gleaming under the soft glow of wall sconces framed by prewar molding. There was the vintage scarf I had found in Paris and had framed, and the 1930s Georgian-inspired bowfront chest of drawers I'd scored at the Grand Bazaar NYC just a few blocks away the decade prior. There was the Moroccan ceramic vase I'd gotten in Fez, the silver tray from a month in Argentina that kept my house keys, and the plush, pale blue sofa that I loved sinking into at the end of the day. There were photos of my four nieces and nephews, and of friends who were chosen family. This wasn't just a nice home that I had made for myself; it was a testament to a life painstakingly curated. I had two degrees, a lucrative and fulfilling career, a grown-up New York City apartment, a dog, and I was house hunting in the Hamptons. I had my shit together.

So, what was *that* just now? A breakdown? A breakthrough?

I had spent the past decade "doing the work" on the therapist's couch. To my knowledge, the shadows of my childhood had been excavated and thoroughly examined. This had been delicate work, scrutinizing the events of my childhood in painful detail. And I was still in therapy, having progressed to spending my weekly sessions on present life matters, which paled in comparison to the childhood stuff I had spent years sifting through. It had never dawned on me that I had not mourned this loss. That I was unconsciously carrying the pain of a lifetime's worth of unspoken sorrows. That this grief was love looking for a home within me, and I had not made space for it.

At seven years old, I witnessed the fragile nature of our existence, and I had no way to understand what I'd experienced—the loss of a parental figure, my grandmother, and my mother's collapse under the weight of grief and crack cocaine. My father nowhere to be found. My young brain enacted a defense mechanism that numbed me to grief's dissonance. While my mother drifted into addiction, I anchored into control, a psychological maneuver that I would learn to repeat, perfect, and execute with strategic precision throughout my life. I allowed Grandma's absence to blur into the background noise. Life moved on and I moved on with it.

Sleep felt far away, and I needed soothing. A walk emerged as the only logical thing to do. I was intent on feeling my weight as I landed each step on the pavement, further evidence that I was not the ghost. At nearly 10:30 p.m., it was too late to walk through the park, so I put on my sneakers, headed the three blocks up Columbus Avenue to 81st Street, and past the American Museum of Natural History toward Central Park West. I tracked the edge of the park, keeping to the west side of the street, where the endless row of doorman buildings offered generous light and a sense of safety. Without my headphones, my thoughts raced, tracing the lines of the evening. *Why had this chosen to surface now? Was it the mere passage of time, or were there other forces at play, orchestrating this emotional reckoning?* Our minds, adept at keeping our emotions balanced, can shroud feelings of loss to prevent overwhelming distress. We build walls to shelter ourselves from the chaos of emotions that threaten to consume us. My own walls had been erected early on, shielding me from the raw pain of loss. Eventually, I had built a fortress. This I had learned from my first therapist, as we explored the extreme mental separation I created from my upbringing to flourish in a more secure life. What I hadn't learned was my body's response. *What do I know that I have forgotten? What else might I have hidden from myself?*

I ambled around my neighborhood until my mind felt clear and my body felt light. Until I walked off an old version of myself. The tears had been cleansing. The cool air, a place of surrender. Drawing a deep breath, I let it mingle with the crisp night before releasing it back into the world, a silent vow to embrace whatever else might come up. As I approached my building, a new hope had grown over whatever the pain of that night had done to me. The image of the car accident became a threshold, a portal urging me to explore greater emotional terrain.

I had found my way back to Grandma. She was leading me somewhere new with the promise that I would find more of myself. I just had to be brave enough to look.

2

FINDING TRUTH
ON THE LIE

I t feels like life should have come to a halt after such time
travel. That evening in my apartment, the past abruptly
tore through the present, a lightning bolt splitting the calm
summer sky. And yet, time remained stubborn and relentless as I remained determined that nothing was wrong. But I
had stumbled blindly, unwittingly, into some piece of myself.
It's the cosmic joke, isn't it? You think you've neatly arranged
life's puzzle pieces, and just as you lean back to admire it, the
Universe nonchalantly flips the table.

What more could I have done? I had survived the worst
things that had ever happened to me and lived to tell the
tale. I now navigated a world of prestige, toting elite degrees
and high-four-figure designer handbags. My tailored blazers
painted a portrait of a chic executive, gracefully command-
ing boardrooms with the winning combination of warmth,

competence, and ambition. Socially, I had many genuine friendships, and my carefully selected acquaintances and hard-to-get invitations into the "right rooms" marked my territory in a sophisticated world.

But the real betrayal I felt came as a result of seeing myself as someone who was known to face and conquer hard things. I took risks and embraced my mistakes. After everything I'd been through, how could something like that go undetected? I took pride in my vigilant self-awareness and willingness to ask probing questions of myself and others. I had done "the work." I had developed a self. I was damn near wellness personified. Yet, in the face of the unsettling discovery of the photo of Grandma's tragic accident, my grace-under-fire self-image, which I had honed to reflect strength and composure, now felt delicate. The sleek design of my life now seemed insufficient to contain the uncharted emotional landscape that lay before me.

I still wonder what led me to search for my grandmother's name that night. Was it that I was a few years away from turning forty? Had an accumulation of milestones—birthdays, breakups, graduations, promotions, and cross-country career moves—triggered the whole thing? I had been on my own for most of these moments, and maybe they had acted as catalysts, awakening something dormant within me. Was I longing for some sort of maternal presence in my life to nurture and guide me, and unaware of it? For most of my life, I had been on a solo mission, fiercely determined to succeed, conquering challenges and clocking the lessons that etched a rich inner world. The life I'd built was proof of my endurance and resilience. No reason to believe otherwise—that would only drag me down.

Seeing that photo of my grandmother's car had broken something wide open in me and threatened to upset my carefully curated life. Suddenly, the world tilted on an unfamiliar axis. I wanted to keep my eyes closed, to shut out the somatic memories that were flooding back with Grandma's ferocity. I tried to cling to the illusion of an unblemished inner life, following the script I'd authored, one that dictated a narrative of triumph over adversity. There was no room for a breakdown or whatever this was. The threat of upheaval would surely leave me in a puddle on the floor. Strangely though, I didn't feel the weight of depression or the nagging grip of anxiety. This was something I couldn't name. And it was more potent than grief. This uninvited emotion demanded acknowledgment, challenging the self-image I had cultivated and grown accustomed to after ten years of therapy: a healed version of myself.

What had I been hiding from myself? And why?

Like an overprotective parent, the brain orchestrates a reality intended to keep us safe from things that might hurt us, a kind of a manufactured amnesia. It was why, in my mind, my mother's drug use had begun after Grandma died. That she was sober and doting before that. That was always how I remembered it, how I remembered her. That was the story I told myself, and later when I could bring myself to talk about it, it was the story I told to others.

I didn't want to remember the night when I was four or five or six and my mother cursed and beat me for telling Grandma that the house had a funny smell when she and her friends were smoking. I don't want to remember how it felt when the back of her hand struck the side of my face and then the top of my head. The way she grabbed my arm so hard, I thought it might release from its socket. Her free hand, open and swift, came down with the weight of her five-foot-seven-inch frame on my back and bare legs. The whiff of cigarettes on her breath and in her hair, the feral vacancy in her eyes.

"You don't tell my motherfucking business! Do you hear me? To nobody! I'm the adult. This is *my* house. I can do what I want."

I don't want to remember the first time I thought my mother might kill me.

We tell ourselves stories to make sense of the senseless, to polish the jagged edges of our painful encounters into a veneer of meaning. We look for the "sermon in the suicide," clinging to a palatable version of reality that makes us feel in control. These narratives give order and purpose to the chaos of our most unimaginable experiences. They allow us to believe that the monsters under the bed have been tamed, and that the demons lurking in our memories have been vanquished. We speak of lessons learned, of wisdom gained, of resilience acquired, as if there is a silver lining to our suffering. We recast our own victimhood as a heroic journey, carving arcs of bravery from despair. Because sometimes, the naked truth, pure and undiluted, is too much to endure. We tell ourselves stories so that we can survive.

This had been a time in my life when I felt a genuine sense of ease. After two years in Providence leading beauty growth strategy and innovation for CVS, I moved back to New York City for my role at Facebook and Instagram, where I worked with luxury beauty and fashion retail brands on their mobile advertising and storytelling strategies on our platforms. Having previously spent nine years in the city, I was happy to be back in the familiar embrace of home. I was once again close to many good friends, even as weddings and babies led some of them to the suburbs. The pulse of the city resonated with me, but so did the call for a bit of respite.

Amid the hustle of working at Facebook and consulting with the incredible Tracee Ellis Ross on what eventually became Pattern Beauty, I realized the city was both my muse and my co-conspirator. The constant inspiration and invigoration are undeniable—to live in NYC is to understand the charge of ambition, to stride with purpose, to learn the staccato rhythm of heels on pavement, the symphony of taxis honking, and the art of brief encounters that linger for days. At the same time, it exhausted me.

"Back in NYC, I see! When can we catch up??" someone would text or email. The second question mark signaled an eagerness to reconnect that I found, at times, flattering. But after one too many invitations to "just catch up" that turned into getting my brain picked for a straight hour, it was time to up the ante on the intention-setting. I needed a filter.

I'd been back for two months when I complained to a friend that I felt overwhelmed by what seemed like unmanageable demand for my energy and underwhelmed by the aftertaste of many of the encounters.

"I'm only saying yes to things that have the potential to make me rich, skinny, or married. In that order," I declared.

She burst into laughter, an affirmation: "Yessss. Love that."

It *was* funny. It was clear, and it landed well. Rich-Skinny-Married quickly became boundary lines. Acquaintances would ask to get together, then joke about whether their requests met my criteria. It turned out to be a reliable filtering mechanism, even if it was a bit crude.

But I had learned my lesson the first time around. I also wanted a place within reasonable driving distance where my soul could stretch, where the rhythm of life could slow to stillness.

I had just started my search for a second home out east, and I dreamed of spending weekdays in the city and weekends on the edge of Long Island, the perfect mix of town and country living. At the end of a week in the city dictated by appointments, errands, and deadlines, heading out east meant a surrender to simplicity. (It's not lost on me that when folks think *Hamptons*, they envision sprawling beachfront mansions and celebrity-studded parties.) But that is not what drew me there. I couldn't even afford to think about buying a tear-down on the water; I was going to get away from people, not party-hop. Even now, I am still much more likely to be found with a glass of wine and a good book or having profound conversations with turkeys and turtles—not exactly the stuff of socialites. I saw such a retreat as a lifeline in a demanding world. My decision to buy a house there would eventually mean more than splitting my time between two places; it would be a venture into living two different lives, each enriching the other. The city urged me to strive. The country, in its quiet wisdom, taught me to be.

Over the years, my love affair with the East End had blossomed. I'd been there in summer share houses with nine other people where we each had a roommate, at weekend gatherings with a friend's aunt and uncle swapping stories in their cozy cottage in the woods, and at my friend Mark's house in Bridgehampton, where we ordered take-out Chinese and discussed the state of the historically Black neighborhoods in Sag Harbor. The allure of the Hamptons was an unspoken promise of tranquility, the feeling of catching your breath in a place that existed outside the chaos of the everyday. I do, admittedly, keep an eye out for Ina Garten every time I go to Citarella, though.

I spent many of my weekends hunting Hamptons real estate, and on my two-hour drives down the Long Island Expressway, I often listened to podcasts, usually ones about women in business, women and wealth, women building things that made life better for others. The Saturday after the weight of mourning for my grandmother had settled, I set off to see a few houses, and during my drive tuned in to a podcast out of my usual league—an episode of the *Guardian's Science Weekly* called "Neuroplasticity: How the Brain Heals." The interview featured Dr. Norman Doidge, a Canadian philosopher turned psychiatrist whose groundbreaking work had helped launch the revolutionary science of neuroplasticity into the mainstream. He had just published his second book, *The Brain's Way of Healing: Remarkable Discoveries and Recoveries from the Frontiers of Neuroplasticity*, in which he shared stories of miraculous recoveries—a man bound by Parkinson's for two decades rediscovering his rhythm, a woman in her sixties banishing inoperable back pain through the power of her own mind. Chronic pain, he argued, is as much a mental condition as a physical one, and there are many mental processing techniques and ways of training the brain that we can use to help alleviate it.

Doidge began with a simple explanation of the concept of neuroplasticity. "Neuro is for neuron, the nerve cells in the brain that fire electrical signals. Plasticity means adaptable, changeable, modifiable." Two minutes into the episode and six miles into my ninety-nine-mile drive, I had to fight the urge to pull over, order both of Doidge's books, and look up everything else that had been written on the topic of neuroplasticity. Instead, I settled in for my very first lesson in neuroscience. "Neuroplasticity is the property of the brain that allows it to change its structure and function in response to activity and mental experience," Doidge explained. "It's the brain's way of doing yoga," I imagined him saying. He was not the first to study or coin the term *neuroplasticity*, but he had popularized it, and with this second book, officially propelled it into the limelight, busting the four-hundred-year-old myth that unlike other parts of the body, the brain can neither regenerate nor heal itself. The brain is not "hard-wired," as it had once been described by the medical community, although its adaptations occur so early in our lives that it often feels that way. Our brains are neither fixed nor predetermined, defying the antiquated notion of the brain as a static, unchangeable organ. Scientists like Doidge and others were presenting cases that proved that the brain's plasticity is a lifelong process and that it is, in fact, fundamental to both brain and mental health throughout our lives.

"You don't have to believe, but you have to be willing to suspend your disbelief," Doidge told the interviewer, who presented the textbook skepticism of a scientist who is also British. She pushed him on the question of clinical trials versus anecdotes of recovery and went on to suggest that Doidge's entire thesis and the more than twenty years of research he drew upon could be reduced to "people's ability to alleviate their symptoms comes down to mental willpower."

"It's not about willpower," he responded. "It's about understanding how the brain works so you can turn on certain switches. There are many dangers that face us as human beings. One danger is that we overstate the role of the mind in helping certain illnesses and conditions. The other danger is that we understate it."

"Oh my God!" I said aloud in response, as if he were talking directly to me.

A doctor was saying what I had somehow long understood. People were harnessing the power of their own minds to overcome obstacles most could never fathom. I felt affirmed, handed the vocabulary to define a practice I had intuitively embraced throughout my life. My survival was not just a random collision of chance; it had been an ongoing exercise in creating from possibility. This was no different from what he was describing in cases of people learning to manage extreme cases of ADHD or to fully function again after debilitating strokes.

"I wish I had known this years ago," I mused, my voice carrying the weight of reflection. Throughout my adult life, sharing the story of my childhood and family background was to ask most people to suspend their disbelief. Upon learning that I was raised in extreme poverty by a single mother whose crippling substance abuse lasted into my adulthood, these people would give me dumbfounded looks, and then, looking more closely as if to seek a trace of the remains, ask: "But how did you know what to do? What drove you? How did you get out and become...*this*?"

These questions hang in the air, wisps of curiosity

tethered to a string of disbelief. *This*, a flourish of the hand sweeping toward me—fingers outstretched, palm open and turned upward, a presentation of the rare and novel. *This*, their voices laced with wonder, their eyes widening in a plea for revelation, for me to provide the link that would bridge the divide between the story of my past and the resolute figure standing before them. The assumption, born from appearances, being that surely, as someone who had graduated college cum laude at the age of twenty from the University of Michigan, who received an MBA from NYU, who at twenty-seven spent a month navigating the streets of Buenos Aires with rusty, 300-level collegiate Spanish, who held an executive role at Facebook after a tour of companies like L'Oréal and Estée Lauder, must have come from privilege, raised in the embrace of a conventional and nurturing family.

To this day, the two questions I am most often asked are some versions of "Do you report the news on TV?" and "Did you do beauty pageants growing up?" To reconcile my origin story with the woman standing before them requires a leap of imagination that few dare to make. Instead, they construct a surrogate backstory that aligns with more "realistic" expectations. A tale built on the myth that only the children of well-educated, industrious, upwardly mobile parents can ascend to the realms of privilege, education, and socioeconomic stability I had reached. A narrative that implied that I could not possibly bear the complexities of such adversity and still create the kind of life to which one usually responds, "Your parents must be so proud." My story defied any expectation of trajectory. The narrative didn't just shift. It shattered.

I could never tell a story about my life in which I was the daughter of a mother enslaved by crack and a father caught in heroin's grip, because this wasn't the story that I told myself. That the monsters in my house weren't under the bed but roaming freely throughout. Even in this truth, even in my existence that stands as my greatest evidence, I know, deep down, that these stories are more than narratives; they are shields we wield against the searing pain of raw recollection. They are also a form of neuroplasticity in action. My story was of a girl who manifested an incredible life because she believed that another life was waiting for her. Mine was a narrative of resilience, yes. I had faced and conquered the unimaginable, my own being as living proof. But these were mere facts about my upbringing, background noise. My story was one of hope, an exploration of belief and conviction, an artistic endeavor of stitching together a life that most people would bet against.

We tell stories about our lives, and if we tell them long enough, our lives become those stories.

What Doidge described—this idea that the brain, ever responsive to our thoughts and actions, can reconfigure, adjust, and reorient itself—was enthralling. As we actively engage in new learning and experiences, the brain's capacity to reorganize and form new neural connections allows it to physically change to accommodate that new information. An artisan of its own becoming, the brain adapts to how we perceive ourselves, our intentions and choices, the ideas we hold dear. This is what is happening in the brain when we listen to a song over and over again until we know every word, every key change, every ad lib. It's the details we rattle off in the exact same way about how we met our best friend or why we chose our dog's name. Or when someone says, "I've always been this way." The more we repeat a behavior or tell ourselves a story, the more potential this story has to become reality—for better or for worse. And it can rescue or ruin us. "If you argue for your limitations you get to keep them," the saying goes. But if we believe that we are destined for something beyond our circumstances, as I had, our brains actually shift and change to help us to achieve it. The concept of neuroplasticity isn't just about reshaping the brain, therefore, but about realizing the innate potential within, the endless adaptability that each of us possesses.

The interview with Doidge was a reckoning and a revelation. It was as if I had been standing in a dark room and suddenly every light came on. Doidge's emphasis on the mind's resilience and adaptability reaffirmed so much of what I thought I knew about my own life. I had carved a path from a devastating childhood, persistently adapting, reshaping, and redefining myself. My ability to persist and evolve, despite my circumstances, was no longer an abstract concept. There was a scientific explanation for it.

Neuroplasticity holds a promise: The stories we tell ourselves about who we are matter, and they can change. These stories, which create a lens through which we view the world, are not fixed. They are mutable and dynamic. They dissolve and reassemble in response to every new space we inhabit, to the people who become our chosen family, to the adventures we pursue, and to the revelatory moments we collect along the way. What we learn we can unlearn. This malleability, I believe, is our greatest gift as humans. To find a new path when the ground shifts beneath us is an invitation. To envision a different way forward is to dream. To continue on after devastating loss might be the truest test of creativity. To write a new story is how we make magic.

If our origin stories hold our power, our ability to rewrite the narrative is our superpower.

As I left the Hamptons, the late autumn sun dipped low, casting a warm glow over the island. I spent the rest of the drive back in contemplation. Surrounded by the ceaseless hum of the highway, I drove in silence for over an hour, thinking about how Doidge's words related to my own story. I had, indeed, penned a new narrative for myself. Amid the wreckage of what once was, the true essence of creativity emerges. When we navigate hardship and survive, we unearth the profound truth that creative living, in its purest form, is not confined to the realm of artists and visionaries. Creativity is the silent revolution that occurs within the human spirit, where the alchemy of endurance transforms adversity into a raw material for the sculpting of a new way to live.

I still believe this. But the deafening crescendo that forced me to confront the thirty-year-old loss of my grandmother would reveal another undeniable truth: The stories we bury, the ghosts we avoid, they dictate our paths without asking for permission. The parts of our stories that we attempt to hide away will eventually come back to haunt us.

As I reached the city, I spotted a bookstore and immediately pulled over. Neither of Doidge's books was in stock there, and I'd have to order them online, but I left with a mission. With the intensity of an investigative journalist, I wanted to immerse myself in the worlds of neuroscience and eventually psychology to understand all that I could about the brain and the mind and the self in order to make sense of my own experience. I would start with Doidge and go from there.

The days that followed were a blur. I went to work, to client meetings, to spin class, to drinks and dinners with friends. The whole time, I kept turning it all over in my mind—the connections between losing Grandma and how the intricate mechanisms of the brain and mind move us toward healing—until I could see my therapist at 7:30 a.m. on Wednesday. It was unusual for me to agree to meet so early and before the workday unfurled, but Norma had come highly recommended by a colleague.

Norma, a Puerto Rican New Yorker, was kind-faced

with a gentle voice, but she had a straightforward way about her that I appreciated. Her proximity to my apartment was a practical consideration and a plus. But what really drew me to her was the kinship I sought—the understanding that could only be forged through our shared experiences of navigating the world as professional women of color. Her own life, a testament to resilience and possibility, unfolded in the few details she shared—marrying in her forties and at forty-eight years old adopting a baby boy who was now in first grade.

I shared the events of the past week with her: stumbling on the photograph of Grandma's accident, unraveling in the wake of its discovery, learning what I had about neuroplasticity, and my insatiable need to make sense of it all.

"I just don't understand why now, after all these years, this would be coming up," I said.

Norma's eyes shifted from her legal pad back to me. "Grief has its own timeline, and it can surface when we least expect it. Your child self did what she needed to survive. Now, it seems your adult self is ready to face what was buried."

A lump formed in my throat as I grappled with the profound truth she presented.

"Yes, but why now? I've spent ten years in therapy at this point." I shifted on the sofa, preparing to plead my defense.

"I've talked about all of this, Norma. I know that we haven't, but *I* have. A lot. I've processed my grandmother's death as a catalyst for how things unfolded in my childhood. I've accepted it and the parents I had or didn't have. And then, I get this sudden urge to look her up and I find the most horrific thing I could have imagined...I just don't get what changed."

She offered an empathetic gaze. "Sometimes, even when we're talking, even when we're analyzing, there are parts of us that stay hidden, waiting for the right moment. Maybe, after all these years, you've reached this place in your life, creating a safe distance from that past, and your psyche deemed you ready." A pause stretched between us. "Perhaps," she continued, "this moment of mourning, arriving as it has, marks not an ending, but a beginning."

3

SEVEN YEARS
OF CHILDHOOD

The more I thought about it that day, the more Norma's comment gnawed at me, refusing to settle into anything meaningful. That night, I tried to distract myself with a book, but her voice kept coming back to me.

"Beginning of what?" I turned it over again in my mind. I was already seven months into a new job and in the early stages of house hunting. I got the sense that these were not the new beginnings she was talking about. The whole thing felt like trying to catch smoke with my bare hands.

I wandered to the kitchen, hoping a cup of tea might help clear my mind. I filled the kettle and set it back on the stove, the familiar click of the gas burner offering a small comfort. As the water heated, I reached for my favorite University of Michigan mug and decaf black tea. I leaned against the counter and stared at the hydrangeas on the dining table.

They were a couple of days old, but their white petals were still crisp, like they'd just been picked, and for a moment, I lost myself in their serenity. The kettle's whistle broke my trance, pulling me back. The simple motions—pouring the boiling water, watching the steam rise, the tea bag bobbing in its brew, adding cream and sugar, stirring it the way I had a thousand times before—brought a brief stillness to my thoughts. I carried the steaming mug back to the living room and sank into the sofa, cradling the warmth in my hands.

I took a small sip, enough for the taste to transport me back to Grandma's kitchen on Hubbell Avenue, a broad, two-lane road lined with rows of unassuming foursquare and bungalow homes common to the American Midwest, built during the mid-nineteenth century. Her house had the kind of Craftsman details that felt sturdy, solid, built to last, even if the years had worn it down. Like the others on her street, Grandma's house was extremely modest, despite its relative proximity to the more esteemed Detroit neighborhoods of Palmer Park and the University District. I imagine that had she not owned three other houses—all inhabited by her adult children—she may have lived in a nicer part of town.

But it felt like pure love. Her warmth was in every corner, every creak of the floors, every worn chair and fading curtain. It filled the space like sunlight spilling in through the windows, soft and steady, turning the ordinary into something sacred. It wasn't about the house itself—it was about the love that lived there. Her love was morning routines that felt like rituals, long weekend breakfasts where she'd cut bananas into my cornflakes, or the sweet smell of scrambled eggs with Bob Evans sausage patties and buttered toast with strawberry or grape preserves. While Grandma savored her coffee, I relished the sweetness of my orange juice.

"Grandma, what does coffee taste like?" I asked the morning after a solo sleepover. I was maybe five.

"Bitter," she answered, adding milk, then sugar.

"Is it good?"

"It's good to grown-ups. You won't like it," she said, stirring. Grandma spoke in short, precise sentences. Her words were few and exact, leaving no room for misinterpretation. Effie Mae Bogard (born Buchanan) wasn't a woman who felt the need to fill silence. She was a serious and hardworking woman born in Okolona, Mississippi, in 1932, at a time when being a Black woman meant facing specific hardships and keeping her indignities to herself. She didn't have to share them for me to know there were many.

I would eventually learn that she married a man who was nine years older and had their first son, Edgar, when she was only fifteen years old. Then came James Isaiah, whom we called Ike, and Frank, spaced just a year apart. Years after her first marriage, she met and married my grandfather. Together, they had my mother, the only girl, and the only child they shared.

"How do you know I won't like it?" I challenged with playful innocence, careful not to speak over her. My eyes fixed on her coffee as it turned the color of my skin.

"Because I know you!" She smiled at me over the top of her glasses. "I'll make you some hot tea. I think you'll like that."

From the cupboard she fetched another white-and-blue floral mug like hers, and a tea bag, and then filled it with hot water. As steam rose, a dark pool began to form, and the tea bag disappeared. Grandma lifted it out and onto a spoon, wrapped the string around it carefully to drain the tea bag, and placed it on a bread plate. Once more, milk, then sugar.

"Can I stir it?" I asked, hopeful, pleading.

"Okay. Keep the spoon all the way down in the mug and go slowly."

My back suddenly as straight as the chair, my open hand ready for my instrument as I took a front-row seat to my own performance. I have since been asked many times if I first discovered English breakfast tea in London. But it was Grandma, who didn't own a passport and who would never travel to Europe, who introduced me to it, right there in her little brown-and-yellow kitchen on Hubbell Avenue. I believe that is what it feels like to be loved. The essential love, unbounded by the constraints of time. The vital love that reassures you that you exist. And that your existence matters.

There are some childhood memories you hold on to, like

that one. Or the first time you rode your bike without training wheels, or the way your mother's eyes lit up when you brought home a drawing from school. And then there are those that, no matter how hard you try, resist the light of understanding. For years, I have struggled to conjure many memories of the before times. Before Grandma died. Before I knew what drugs were and that my mother couldn't stop using them. I try to remember images of her before everything changed, a bit of something, like sitting in her lap or her bandaging my scraped knee. Nothing comes to me. I find myself trying to go back, to revisit the corridors of my past, but the doors remain locked, and the keys seem misplaced. I was too young to remember the days before the drugs took hold, her laughter a rare sound that faded more each year. My first memories hold little recollection of a time when my mother's presence wasn't tinged with acute anger or distant sorrow. I am locked out of the before times. Some of that seems intentional, a deliberate forgetting. My body has learned the art of shielding me from my own mind. It knows when to step in, preventing me from settling into cruel, unloving reminiscence and keeping me from straying too far from my center. Some memories are better left out of reach.

It seems telling, then, that my most vivid memory from that time is marked by the afternoon that I ran away from home. My mother was upstairs asleep in her bedroom, leaving me to entertain myself with the television. I don't remember where Leah was, but the *Thundercats* kept me company. After the show ended, I went upstairs to use the bathroom, after which, in the manner of curious six-year-olds, I decided to test just how powerful the toilet was. I proceeded to unroll the toilet paper and fill the toilet until all of the water had been absorbed.

And then I flushed it.

Before I knew it, the bowl had filled up around the mound of soaked tissue, and within moments I was standing in an inch of water. Unsure of what to do next, I ran downstairs, where I realized that the water was leaking through the bathroom floor into the kitchen. I was going to have to do the scariest thing I could imagine in that moment: wake my mother from her nap. I tiptoed quickly into her room, hoping to preserve her final moments of peace before ruining her day. I shook her gently, until she opened her eyes and lifted her head toward me. I told her about the flood, holding out hope that this news would be met with understanding, comfort, and swift problem-solving.

She leaped from the bed and into the hallway, where the carpet was now also getting soaked.

"Daria!" She sprinted to the bathroom to find my crime scene. Her eyes darted from the overflowing toilet to the spreading water to the towel bar and finally settled on me, wide-eyed and trembling in the hallway. I could see the transformation in her face, a swift shift from grogginess to a blazing fury that could only mean one thing.

"What the fuck did you do?" she shouted, her voice echoing off the walls.

I shrank back toward the stairs, my heart pounding in my chest. "I didn't mean to do it, I was just trying to see if I could flush the tissue."

"You didn't mean to?" she mocked me, her anger only growing. "You meant it just like I'm going to mean it when I beat your ass!"

I spent no time contemplating my fate. I had learned early on to fear her temper and that fear drove me straight out the front door and onto my bike, which I'd only learned the year before to ride without training wheels. I rode my bike past my classmate Shanise's house, but her parents' car wasn't in the driveway, so I kept going, down Dawes Street and onto Joy Road—a busy main street in Northwest Detroit—and then two miles to my uncle Ike's house, taking the route I'd seen Grandma drive many times before.

But when I got to the house, he wasn't home. I sat on the porch for a few minutes, plotting my next move.

"You okay?" a neighbor across the street yelled out. Maybe I'd been sitting for more than a few minutes, long enough to raise concern.

"Yes, I was just waiting for my uncle Ike," I said, reasoning with the obvious absurdity that I was clearly there alone.

Having raised suspicion, I knew I needed to relocate. It then dawned on me that my dad's parents lived down the street. I hopped on my bike and rode the two blocks to my other grandparents' house. Surely someone would be home. My dad was one of nine children and there were already at least ten grandchildren by that time. Someone was always at that house, whether they lived there or not.

At first, my grandmother Thelma smiled when she realized it was me at the door. I felt relief. But it was quickly squashed when her smile was overrun by confusion and concern.

"Daria? What...What are you doing here?"

"By herself?" my grandfather chimed in, moving toward us as I entered the front door.

"This child rode her bike," Grandma Thelma said.

"Daria! Did you really ride your bike all the way over here?" Grandad said, needing confirmation.

"Where are you coming from?" Grandma Thelma doubled down.

I sobbed my story until she put me down for a nap. I awoke to learn my mother had been informed of my whereabouts and that I would be promptly taken home.

It's all there, stored with great clarity, even the moment that my bike was stowed in the back of my grandparents' station wagon as the sun was setting and I in the back seat. Everything that happened after is gone. I don't remember anything that happened after I had been returned to my rightful place of residence—what my mother said or did. It says a lot that I was less afraid of running away than staying.

I want to ascribe it to childhood amnesia, the phenomenon where early memories remain shrouded in forgetfulness, a byproduct of the rapid development of the brain during those formative years. The brain, in its swift growth, sculpts neural connections, relegating most early memories to the shadows of implicit recall. It's growing so quickly, in fact, that although we begin to form conscious memories at around two and a half years of age, most memories—save the ones that stick—elude conscious recall until around the age of seven.

But somehow, I remember the pets we had before Grandma died: Rusty, the German shepherd who was a welcome member of the family until he knocked a toddling Leah down in the front yard and tore her coat. Then there was Cocoa, a sweet little Bouvier like Grandma's dog, Champ, who suddenly got sick and died. I even vaguely remember the white rabbits that lived in a cage in Uncle Frank's garage. Mostly, I remember being told that a neighborhood dog found and ate them. Still, I often find myself trying to work out whether a lapsed memory is a result of this peculiar realm of childhood, or whether the many blank spots of my early life are a result of the ways in which I became separated from the abnormalities of mine specifically.

Those first seven years of our lives are the most crucial for development, making them a time of great potential and great vulnerability. The brain is completing its most important work, laying the foundation for future growth and shaping the structure of our initial sense of being. During this time, the brain is a veritable construction site, building and wiring and forming connections at a rapid pace.

Even before birth, during the third trimester, the senses begin to stir. Our mother's voice, her scent, the food she eats—they all start to register. By the time we're born, her voice and smell are already imprinted into our consciousness, easing our transition from the womb to the world. In just a few short months, we become adept at eliciting caregiving, responding to faces, voices, and sounds. Before age three, our brains are creating a dizzying one million neural connections a minute. By five, 90 percent of your brain development is done; the neuro-architectural structure has largely been built. And just like any construction project, the materials and the workmanship that go into building the structure will determine its strength and durability. They establish whether that structure—our mind, our sense of self—will be strong enough to weather whatever comes next.

We enter the world primed to connect with our mothers—our infant brains are wired this way. We are biologically designed for attachment, and it's essential for our survival, in both a physical and emotional sense. As infants, we also quickly become acquainted with and learn to adapt to the subtle ways in which our mothers, fathers, and other caregivers show up to meet our needs, or don't. How and when we're fed, the amount of time we are left to cry before we're held or changed, the generosity or lack of attention and quality of time that we receive—these things are wired into our brains. In a few short months, our little minds start forming patterns, responding to the warmth or neglect in our environment. For the adults, especially in those attuned to care for a baby, those signals evoke an instinct to nurture and protect.

If the mother is overwhelmed with stress and anxiety, she is unable to serve as a "container" for the child's own anxieties and aggressions. D. W. Winnicott, a renowned psychoanalyst who also practiced as a pediatrician, emphasized the crucial role of a mother's emotional state in shaping a child's development. In his view, the mother's ability to provide a sense of security for the child is essential. "The mother's initial holding environment is vital because the infant is completely dependent on the mother's containing of its anxieties and aggressions. If a mother is anxious and stressed herself, she will not be able to provide this containing function and the infant's sense of security will be damaged. This can lead to difficulties later in life in dealing with frustration and in establishing relationships."

In an ideal world, a child has two loving, present, emotionally regulated parents who are bolstered by resources and strong support systems. Mama had Grandma, that was clear. And somehow, as much as my mother's, Grandma's presence is a constant woven into the fabric of those early years. I have since wondered what I miscarried for lack of observation from Grandma. For lack of being seen by her. "There wasn't enough time," I thought. "I wish I'd known that I needed to write it all down," I scribbled in my journal. I feel a kind of greed, a desperate longing for something more to remember her by, something beyond the image of her death. Something more than my mind gives me access to.

When our roots are torn, the earth beneath us feels like it might give way, leaving us suspended in an unknowable space. Early childhood trauma, abuse, and neglect carve deep grooves into our tender psyches, and the nervous system becomes a vigilant watchdog standing guard against any threats, real or imagined. Trauma changes the brain, and the younger we are when we experience it, the deeper and more potentially lasting its imprint. The loss of a parental figure compounds this, creating a void where there should have been solace and guidance, shaping the way we see the world and our place in it.

Childhood, when it is lost, is nothing like the haphazard way we misplace our keys or forget names. It's a vanishing act, not performed with a flourish, but with a quiet untethering from safe naivete. There is no grand stage for the disappearance of the child self, no audience to witness the subtle transformation into something fractured and more knowing. Childhood, when it is taken, leaves behind an emptiness that echoes with the absence of what should have been. The theft is a quiet one, a pilfering of laughter and of wonder, replaced by the weight of adult concerns. There is no memorial service laying the child self to rest. Instead, the burial is the result of a quiet erosion of self that takes place in the moments between daylight and dusk.

What I felt in the instance of my grandmother's death and my mother's neglect was sadness, fear, confusion, deprivation, and wanting—for nurturance, guidance, protection, for things I didn't know I needed, for my inability to acknowledge let alone communicate those needs. I came to understand it as an acceleration of the inevitable. We all grow up sometime.

I don't crave anything from that time. There's nothing I can remember wanting to relive. When I picture myself as a little girl, there is no nostalgia in the recollection. No sentimental longing for being tucked in at night, or for the birthday party where we went to the pumpkin patch, or for summer vacations where I was taught to swim. There is only the wistful ache for the little girl who was forced to grow up too fast. I remember the face of my first-grade teacher, Mrs. Messisco, when she overheard me telling a classmate that there was a "bad" word in the title of the Dick and Jane series that we were reading in class. Her expression was one of astonishment, as she asked me to repeat myself and to point out the forbidden word. I complied, unwilling to say it, even though she explained that Dick was the boy's name and that it was a common nickname for Richard. She sent a note home with me that day, informing my mother of the incident and expressing her concern that a child my age was familiar with such language. There was no punishment awaiting me when I got home; I don't even remember there being a conversation about it. And I had learned not to tell Grandma.

I was the girl who, at ten, would call 911 after finding her mother unconscious in bed one afternoon and watch EMTs take her away in an ambulance. My mother all but shrugged it off. "It was due to a minor respiratory issue," she explained, even though she had to be kept overnight. Not long after that, I would find her passed out topless on her bed with the crack pipe still in her hand. I walked over to her and put my finger under her nose to check for her breath and studied her chest to watch it slowly rise and fall before pulling the blanket over her.

Being hailed as a survivor of childhood abuse has always stirred an unsettling ache within me. Everyone loves to celebrate the survivor. What no one acknowledges is that it is a heavy label to wear, the burden of its weight almost unbearable at times. What they don't tell you is that survival has a metallic taste to it, slow and leaden, like blood on the tongue. The air grows thick with memories you'd rather forget, and it has a smell, a mixture of scents that should never coexist, like a field of roses tainted by the scent of a burning body. Any attempt to speak it requires the complex combination of consonants and vowels, the perfect articulation and control of airflow. And all too easily, the syllables get stuck in your throat, a choked elegy for the innocence that once was.

For all the celebration of survival, no one tells you to account for its cost. How survival, in its honorable relentless march forward, is not synonymous with wholeness. We don't survive whole. We move on without acknowledging that some parts of ourselves are too delicate for a new beginning. Thrust into an involuntary act of invention, we will fathom and then forge a new life from the fragments that endure. We talk about growing up and moving on, but seldom do we talk about the remains left in the wake of a premature ending. There is no warning that the road to reinvention is littered with the debris of the former self that we shed.

What did I leave behind?

In *Emotional Inheritance*, Galit Atlas, PhD, explores "intergenerational transmission," where unresolved issues of parents or even distant ancestors can imprint on their descendants' emotional lives. She notes, "The secrets of the mind include not only our own life experiences but also those that we unknowingly carry with us: the memories, feelings, and traumas that we inherit from previous generations." Children may inherit not just the psychological consequences of living with addicted parents but also the unresolved emotional issues that may have contributed to their addiction in the first place. *What did I carry with me? How much of it is even mine?*

Before this awakening, I had little interest in revisiting, or attempting to quantify, the ordeals of my childhood. It seemed like an unproductive exercise and, frankly, an unappealing way to live. I believed that analyzing the past was only helpful inasmuch as it could inspire my future. Spend too much time there, though, and you will get stuck. I felt fully aware of how the ghosts of my past showed up at times in my work and in relationships. Through years of therapy and a lot of hard work, I believed that I had developed an effective toolkit for mitigating their effects. I had never once considered the potential impact of trauma on our hormones, our immune systems, or how it informs the way our DNA is read and expressed. That is, until I began to learn about what really happens when we experience trauma and the ways in which we can use neuroplasticity for healing.

I went from Norman Doidge to Joe Dispenza and Dr. Leah Swart, then to Bessel van der Kolk and Judith Lewis Herman. I found Bruce Perry and Gabor Maté. I turned to Carl Jung and discovered the work of Nadine Burke Harris, former surgeon general of California and, to my misfortune, no known relation. They, and many others, would become my teachers, helping me to understand the road that I'd traveled, and illuminating a path forward. Collectively, their research, writing, and practice would be my introduction to psychological fields of study such as epigenetics and the impact of childhood trauma on brain development and long-term health and well-being.

In her 2014 TED Talk, Burke Harris spoke of the 1995 CDC–Kaiser Permanente study on adverse childhood experiences (ACEs), one of the largest investigations on the impact of childhood abuse and neglect on health and well-being later in life. Child psychiatrists who specialize in the study of ACEs theorize that the more ACEs a person has, the more likely that person is to experience physical, mental, and/or social health problems as an adult. The two-year study also suggests that exposure to six or more ACEs can lower an individual's life expectancy by nearly twenty years.

The ACE study identified the ten events that are most likely to rewire the brain based on their traumatic effect. The loss of a parent or close caregiver is categorized as an ACE. At age two, I'd lost my father through my parents' separation. Just after my seventh birthday, as my own sense of identity was beginning to form, I experienced two more devastating losses: my grandmother to death and my mother to grief, depression, and addiction. After watching Burke Harris's talk, I knew that I had to take the ACE test, though I feared what it would tell me.

Before your eighteenth birthday...

Did a parent or other adult in the household often or very often...swear at you, insult you, put you down, or humiliate you? Or act in a way that made you afraid that you might be physically hurt?

Did a parent or other adult in the household often or very often...push, grab, slap, or throw something at you? Or ever hit you so hard that you had marks or were injured?

Did an adult or person at least five years older than you ever...touch or fondle you or have you touch their body in a sexual way? Or attempt or actually have oral, anal, or vaginal intercourse with you?

Did you often or very often feel that... no one in your family loved you or thought you were important or special? Or your family didn't look out for each other, feel close to each other, or support each other?

Did you often or very often feel that...you didn't have enough to eat, had to wear dirty clothes, and had no one to protect you? Or your parents were too drunk or high to take care of you or take you to the doctor if you needed it?

Was a biological parent ever lost to you through divorce, abandonment, or other reason?

Was your mother or stepmother: often or very often pushed, grabbed, slapped, or had something thrown at her? Or sometimes, often, or very often kicked, bitten, hit with a fist, or hit with something hard? Or ever repeatedly hit over at least a few minutes or threatened with a gun or knife?

Did you live with anyone who was a problem drinker or alcoholic, or who used street drugs?

Was a household member depressed or

mentally ill, or did a household member attempt suicide?

Did a household member go to prison?

With one point for each "yes," I have an ACE score of nine. Neither of my parents were imprisoned; both have been to jail. By age eleven, I had experienced nearly every kind of household dysfunction and emotional disruption that this research indicates would increase my likelihood of smoking, abusing alcohol or drugs, and engaging in risky sexual behavior, and would lead to poor physical and mental health as an adult.

People with an ACE score of seven or more, the study tells us, have three and a half times the risk of heart disease, the leading cause of death in the United States for more than a hundred years. Burke Harris notes how an ACE score of four or more "impact[s] the developing brains and bodies—areas like the pleasure and reward center of the brain" and "inhibits the prefrontal cortex, which is necessary for impulse control and executive function and critical for learning." In the face of what it perceives to be a traumatic event, the brain's command center for focus, concentration, decision-making, and emotional regulation is being stifled while the limbic system, whose job is to detect and respond to threats, amplifies the fear response, leading to a heightened state of anxiety and hypervigilance. "Children are especially vulnerable," Burke Harris warns, "because their bodies are [still] developing. Such toxic stress impacts their neurological, immune, and hormonal systems."

ACE scores are cautionary, however, not predictive. My ACE score of nine doesn't consider the close, loving relationship I had with Grandma for the first seven years of my life; or the teachers who believed in and supported me through my early years, like Ms. Suber, my second-grade teacher, who, on a Saturday, offered to take me and Leah to see *Snow White* during its fiftieth-anniversary release in theaters and then to McDonald's for Happy Meals. It doesn't account for my innate propensity to thrive, or for the nearly twenty years of internal work I've done as an adult.

Childhood trauma is not a life sentence.

4

SEE. BELIEVE. BECOME.

B y the time I was eight, leaving Detroit felt like my destiny. Even then, I saw it as a place of little imagination
or faith, the irony being that there was a church at the end of
our block. But I don't mean religious faith. I mean the kind
of faith that a poor Black girl in a poor Black city needed to
shape her own fate. Somehow, I found room enough inside
myself to nurture a deep curiosity about the world and my
place in it. I clung to any image that suggested there was
a world beyond Detroit, something waiting for me past the
borders of my imagination. Children don't have wisdom or
experience. They have imagination. And anything can happen in a daydream.

In my daydreams, I lived in a world that I had created
for myself, one that promised safety, happiness, and limitless
possibility. In the cramped space on the floor between the
sofa and the TV stand where I would sketch, color, and lose

myself in books, I gathered the materials to build the life I was meant to live. I could close my eyes and escape the reality of our empty fridge, the moldy smell in the basement that flooded with every heavy rain, and the security bars on all the windows that made the house look like a cage. I can still picture the mini fashion magazine I created from folded notebook paper. On each page, I drew models in different outfits, their names carefully rendered in big block letters across the bottom. I described their clothes in great detail, each creation carrying me farther from the constraints of our eight-hundred-square-foot house.

I envisioned a future where I was a successful, independent woman. I could see it so clearly—my brownstone in New York City, just like the Huxtables, and a beach house in Los Angeles like Malibu Barbie. I'd imagine myself driving to work and walking into an office. In business meetings and at dinner parties. And then I would tell Leah all about it with the same level of detail, building on my vision with each round. I never believed in the tooth fairy. I stopped believing in Santa in second grade. The Easter Bunny never stood a chance. I believed in Clair Huxtable and Dominique Deveraux. I still do.

Those women were my magnifiers, reflections of the future I yearned for. They embodied everything I sought to manifest—strength, intelligence, creativity, security, and freedom—giving my brain a model for what was possible. One of the brilliant things that happens when you allow yourself to visualize a different reality is that you begin to pattern your thoughts and mental processes, a phenomenon known as imagery training. In our subconscious minds, where imagination resides, we don't distinguish between past, present, and future, between dream and reality. In fact, the more vividly we dream, the more our minds have to draw upon to forge our reality.

There's a difference between believing something and *knowing* it. Belief can be fragile, a wispy thing that can be shaken in the face of serious doubt. It is an act of hope, a casting forward into the unknown. I am big on belief. But *knowing* is something else. Knowing is rooted someplace deep and untouchable, a bone-deep certainty that stands unyielding even when the world trembles. Belief asks for assurance; knowing asks for nothing. If I believed in a world beyond Detroit, it was on a fourth-grade field trip that I came to truly know it.

As the school bus wound its way toward the Detroit Institute of Arts, I sat in breathless wonder, my eyes fixed on its marble Beaux Arts facade. The rest of the city slipped into obscurity as I was transported to another world. Mr. Lewis, my fourth-grade teacher who led the field trip, stood at the front of the bus beaming. "The Detroit Institute of Arts is home to one of the world's most significant art collections," a point of pride that he wanted us to share. His smile insisted that it belonged to all of us.

A cast of Rodin's *The Thinker* awaited us at the museum's

entrance. The sculpture seemed to be inviting us to join him in quiet reflection as we disembarked.

"What do you think he's thinking 'bout?" I heard a voice say from a few rows behind me.

"Probably who took his clothes!" a boy cracked, punctuated by a chorus of laughter.

As we crossed the threshold into the atrium of the museum, we were reminded to listen to the docent, to take in everything, and to touch nothing. How could I dream of touching anything in this place? I was gripped by awe: the columns and cornices, the spiral staircase descending into a medieval banquet hall that convinced me we had wandered into a castle. The grand halls and gilded frames spoke of a world that was both ancient and immediate, experiences that somehow existed then and continued into now. The artists whose work we discovered spanned the globe: Matisse from France, van Gogh from the Netherlands, Diego Rivera from Mexico, and Berber textiles from Morocco—countries I would one day visit and love. Each piece of art was a tribute to lives that had existed—vivid, curious, enduring—far beyond our history lessons.

That day at the DIA, a portal opened for me, and I peered into it. The short glimpse was long enough to awaken in me the desire to experience the world beyond Detroit. It became a map, a way to navigate the uncharted territories of my future, teaching me that the world was vast and that I was destined to explore its many facets. I wanted to be out *there.* I vowed to make the world my home. I spent the next nine years with my eyes fixed on the horizon, looking ahead to my departure. Eventually, I applied to and was accepted by the University of Michigan, where I completed my undergraduate studies. From there, I left the state to embark on my life, only returning once or twice a year to visit my sister and her kids.

Still, in 2017, I was unnerved to learn that Uncle Frank had sold my childhood home. Just months before, I had visited Leah and the kids, and the thought never crossed my mind that selling the house had even been discussed. I could have offered to buy the house, if only to keep it in the family. Grandma had bought the duplex some time before I was born; Mama, Leah, and I lived on one side, and Uncle Frank and Aunt Pam lived on the other. If I had known, I would have at least wanted to see it one last time.

I imagined calling Leah, demanding answers. "Why didn't you tell me that Uncle Frank sold the house?" I'd ask.

"Yeah, he sold it at the end of last year," she'd reply, almost dismissively.

"Yes, I know. Nikki told me. I'm asking why *you* didn't tell me."

"Why? Did you want it?"

"Maybe. I just hate that it's no longer in the family. It's like there's officially nothing left. And it sold for only twenty-two thousand five hundred dollars?! That's practically nothing." I felt sick.

"Girl, whatever. When was the last time you even talked to Uncle Frank? Or seen that house?"

And she would have been right. I had been estranged from my parents for fifteen years. Detroit had been the place I blamed for almost everything. I could barely stand to be back there. It felt easier to direct my anger toward the city than to the adults who'd failed to care for me while I lived there. Confronting the details of Grandma's accident had put a spotlight on everything I had lost. Now, the house I grew up in, the last of the four she once owned and had left to my mom and uncle, was gone too. It felt like losing a piece of myself, a root severed. I had no family stories, the kind you rehearse until they feel like part of you. The kind you hear so often that even the memories that don't belong to you start to feel like they might be yours. Once Grandma died, no one in my family had bothered taking up the mantle of keeping those stories alive. This should have been my first clue that maybe there wasn't much to hold on to.

For years after leaving, I struggled to remember much about the city and my time there. My memories were somehow trapped, roaming about the rooms I once lived in. But knowing that the house was gone, I suddenly had the urge to revisit them, to see what they might have to tell me. Rooms are witnesses to our lives, keepers of our stories. Time capsules that hold layers of our history and identity. They speak not just of who we were, but of who we hoped to become. The light we choose to let in, the way we arrange our belongings, what we keep and what we throw away—all of it tells a story. *What was my story if I didn't have access to any of this?*

I grew up on Ohio Street, in the northwest part of town, our house one in a line of redbrick duplexes, each with white-trimmed windows and porch railings. There was an uninspired uniformity to our block, which was offset mostly by the occasional missing shutter, left without its twin. The street itself was unremarkable, other than the grassy median that ran down its center with oak trees planted like tent-poles, a small pocket of green in a city grappling with its own decay and a nod to the suburban ideal that Detroit once aspired to. My mother called it a boulevard, a name I liked for its elegance, even if it was a misnomer. The medians reminded me of two of Detroit's actual boulevards, named for Martin Luther King Jr. and Rosa Parks, with their rows of dilapidated buildings and abandoned homes, remnants of failed retail and residential projects. Whenever we drove down them, it struck me as ironic that no one had taken better care of them given their namesakes.

In justifying my own outmigration, I reckoned that there were two types of Detroiters: those who never leave, and those who break free and never look back, a bifurcation meant to say as much about resilience and human potential as it says about the way the places we inhabit inform our identities, and how we get stuck. Those who stayed, I rationalized, had somehow missed the pull of their potential. I interpreted their entrenchment as loyalty at best and complacency at worst. By contrast, those of us who left never to return did not share this blind loyalty to the city. We had seen the worst of it, and we would not be sticking around to test our fate, our determination to succeed masquerading as common sense.

The Detroit I'd grown up in was a city grappling with its past and uncertain about its future. It had once been an economic powerhouse and center of cultural innovation, the beating heart of 1.8 million lives. But time hadn't been good to her, and she was no longer good for her people. I was raised amid its ruins; no one from my old neighborhood had wealth or the clear promise of a brighter tomorrow. Some had religion. But most just had a long list of problems: ailing parents to care for, too many mouths to feed, bills piling up faster than the checks came in. I remember feeling like everything in the city was broken—the school system, the job market, the pavement on the freeways, the windows on every empty house and building. Souls rendered blind. It was easy for me to decide that anything good that would come from the city had to leave in order to thrive. Your dreams could be born in Detroit, but if you stayed, they would die there. This may be the greatest irony of the twentieth century, given Detroit's role in the making of the American Dream.

Once the fourth-largest and the richest city in the United States, the Detroit of today has yet to fully recover from the 1967 Uprising, recorded by the Detroit Historical Society as the largest civil disturbance of twentieth-century

America. Over the course of five days in July 1967, dozens of people tore through the one-hundred-block area of the Virginia Park neighborhood, leaving nearly four hundred people dead or injured, with some fourteen hundred buildings destroyed by fire, amassing fifty million dollars in damages, and leaving an estimated five thousand people homeless. Comparable to a full-scale natural disaster, the true loss and devastation are incalculable, with aftershocks that would be felt for decades. A community left hanging in the balance. Between abundance and lack. Fear and revolt. Mania and unmoving clarity. A West African proverb warns us: "The child who is not embraced by his village will burn it down just to feel the warmth."

The riots were the culmination of decades of racial discrimination, giving rise to a psychological heat wave that burst into flame in the dog days of summer. Even more than New York, Chicago, and Philadelphia, Detroit once offered the promise of prosperity to European immigrants and to citizens from the American South, both Black and white, traveling northward during the Great Migration. In the fifteen-year span from 1944 to 1959, when my mother was born, the city of Detroit saw a shift toward Black wealth, with the proportion of Blacks living in poverty plunging from 85 percent to 55 percent. Still, many Black Americans who chose to relocate in search of a brighter future found that they were weighed down by the structural racism of Reconstruction and Jim Crow. The idea that Black Americans were entitled to the same opportunities in Detroit as their white counterparts, or that they might have parity in their line of sight, was both a threat to and a promise of the institution of American capitalism, a concept too fragile to sustain with the rise of oil prices and competition from foreign car manufacturers.

When progress inspires political backlash, the safest recourse may be to shrink away, seeds of vitality shriveling atop scorched earth. The alternative? Detour from the high road and burn the motherfucker down. Birmingham, 1963. Los Angeles, 1965. Chicago, 1966. Tampa, Cincinnati, Newark, 1967. One week later, Detroit. The fractures had become fault lines.

More than a decade before the 1967 Uprising, Detroit's mayor Albert Cobo and other local policy decision-makers determined that the city needed a complete redesign to keep white people from leaving and to draw now-suburban former residents back to the city, along with a freeway to help them get there. Having been declared slums, Detroit's Black Bottom and Paradise Valley neighborhoods were razed, and architect Ludwig Mies van der Rohe was commissioned to design Lafayette Park, the largest collection of buildings he'd develop in his esteemed career. By most measures, Lafayette Park was deemed a success and became a template for other urban renewal efforts around the country, even as the rest of the neighborhoods surrounding it had been bulldozed and fully vacated. With only thirty days' notice, the residents of

Black Bottom and Paradise Valley were displaced with no help from the government. Their fates served as yet another reminder that racism was not, in fact, confined to the South. The "lucky" ones got to move to one of two public housing projects. The mayor got Cobo Hall and Cobo Arena named after him.

A line had been drawn.

There had been no history lessons on how we got there, no recognition of the role generational neglect had played in the Detroit I had grown up in, no making sense of why our points of pride rested on things long gone. Virtually nothing of the previous life of these neighborhoods has been preserved. Only the echoes of industry ingrained in the concrete, the scars of struggle etched into the streets. Even the most inspired mind would struggle to imagine the cultural community that had once thrived on land now paved over by I-75, as you drive past Whole Foods and Comerica Park. I have tried. Paradise Theatre was eventually restored after standing a vacant, decaying monument for twenty years. Its seven-million-dollar renovation came with a new name, Orchestra Hall, but I'm grateful it remains. Still, I always leave with the same question: Who gets to decide what is worthy of redemption?

By contrast, Detroit's Renaissance Center, a foolhardy corporate attempt to resurrect the city birthed in the 1970s under the premise of "if you build it, they will come." Seven connected commercial high-rise buildings stood for decades as an homage to a city long gone. Each tower, a totem of unmet potential. The megastructure, bearing the ironic name of a city that would take forty years to show any signs of a possible rebirth. That Detroit was more of an idea by then. Henry Ford and the other masterminds of the Renaissance Center had failed to grasp the ways in which decades of decline and desolation had restructured the DNA of Detroit. Below the surface there were forces at work, shaping the city in ways unseen. With every business that closed, every job that was lost, a collective depression grew. Despondence flowed slow and deep like tar pouring out to form a new road, one that passed abandoned factories and storefronts and into neighborhoods, pervading the psyche of nearly everyone who inhabited the city. It became a social contagion with a blast radius that seemed to impact the city's then 1.2 million residents, passed on through bloodlines. Detroit's hopelessness was epigenetic, paving over generational dreams and leading to dead ends. This was the legacy of those left behind. It wasn't just on the surface; it was marrow deep.

If Detroit couldn't recover from such devastation and destruction, I wondered, how could I possibly stay and recover from my childhood? Low self-worth seemed to be a way of living where I came from, and the reward for settling was fitting in. Only now am I able to consider the cognitive load, the invisible weight that the poverty and violence surrounding me imposes on the brain.

The greatest nuisance of human existence might be that

we are hardwired to seek out and trust the familiar, even when the familiar isn't safe or good for us. Trauma halts our capacity to imagine what could be, to learn from new experiences, and to grow. For children, the impact can be lifelong. As Bessel van der Kolk says, "The brains of traumatized kids develop in a 'use-dependent' manner—they become experts in dealing with threat, and have problems with self-regulation, play, and the sort of imaginative creativity that is necessary to become productive members of society."

The architecture of the brain responds to the environment in which it resides, a testament to the organ's malleability. The brain, bent by the gravitational pull of lack, reshapes its contours and its priorities to navigate limited resources. "Entitlement," journalist Andrea Elliott writes in *Invisible Child*, "is born of self-worth. Some people have it naturally. Others must develop it against the proof of their experience." We are hardwired for hope, but belief takes practice. For those of us born into struggle, this becomes impossible unless we are in an environment that nurtures our growth.

I now understand why someone might wonder, "Why hope for something you have no real chance of receiving?" When you grow up surrounded by poverty, abuse, and violence—at home, in school, in your neighborhood—it's not uncommon to accept your circumstances as commonplace, even expected. A multiplicity of stressful forces that become so ordinary, they fail to register as traumatic events.

The repeated exposure results in an emotional sedation from which you may never fully awake.

Surviving under such conditions puts a constant, draining demand on both body and mind. Each day stretches the limits of your endurance, siphoning your energy as if simply making it through is a battle you fight over and over again. The weight of this exhaustion is invisible, but it's there in the way your body tenses, in the sleepless nights, in the feeling of being caught in a cycle that leaves no room for rest or reflection.

The State of Poverty is governed by its own set of rules, an unwritten code that its inhabitants internalize deeply. Those who dwell there must numb themselves to the ceaseless demands of merely existing, a constant hum of survival that overrides all else. In this place, the lack of resources bends time itself, distorting it, speeding it up with the urgency to secure today's sustenance. Time compresses under the weight of need, shrinking, leaving little mental space for thoughts beyond the desperate and immediate. This urgency leads to a kind of tunnel vision, where survival becomes a relentless drama.

In this drama, the brain, molded by the forces of environment and experience, turns its focus inward. The aperture narrows to the present moment, obscuring potential dreams and possibilities. The sharp edges of want blur any vision of the future, making it difficult to see beyond the pressing needs of now. For those in this state, a dream is just another luxury item priced beyond reach. There is only an either/or because "yes, and" costs too much. Choices become binary in the face of scarcity. The State of Poverty enforces a brutal pragmatism. You learn to calculate every risk, to measure every possibility against the hard limits of your reality.

Unnamed trauma is still trauma. And it changes us. Only in my lifetime has research begun to reveal what intergenerational trauma does to the brain and the body, and how we might inherit it from our parents, and their parents. When it comes to the effects of trauma, both nature and nurture play a role. The National Institutes of Health (NIH) reports that "trauma can leave a chemical mark on a person's genes, which can then be passed down to future generations. This mark doesn't cause a genetic mutation, but it does alter the mechanism by which the gene is expressed. This alteration is not genetic, but epigenetic." In other words, trauma doesn't change your DNA, but the traumatic event is an external force that sits on top of your genes, changing whether certain traits are expressed and, therefore, how you behave. And environment matters—it can define whether the traumatic incident will accelerate one's genetic propensity to experience adverse mental health effects or succumb to addiction, or whether it will merely register as distressing but without lasting impact. A genetically predisposed person who grows up in an environment where their physical and emotional needs are met becomes far less likely to develop PTSD after a potentially traumatizing experience, or to seek relief at the bottom of a bottle of gin. From our diet to our exposure to toxic chemicals to our social circles, our environments, and our relationship to them, will either feed us or deplete us. They play the most critical role in who and how we are.

Despair, therefore, is a habit. And fear is highly contagious. So is rage...

"What happened? Why did it happen? What can be done to prevent it from happening again?" These were the questions President Lyndon Johnson posed to the Kerner Commission, an advisory group he assembled to report on the root cause of the short but catastrophic string of riots and propose a way forward to a "decent and orderly society in America." The commission led a seven-month landmark study on race, inequality, and policing, and in 1968 the four-hundred-plus-page Kerner Commission Report was published. Their clear, unwavering thesis in summary: *Our Nation is moving toward two societies, one black, one white—separate and unequal. Reaction to last summer's disorders has quickened the movement and deepened the division. Discrimination and segregation have long permeated much of American life; they now threaten the future of every American.*

No response, not even from the president, who commissioned the report and handpicked the politically moderate, mostly white task force to lead it. Deafening silence. Incessant injustice. Fuel for the emotional inheritance of neglect. The 1955 leveling of Black Bottom and the lack of affordable housing made available to the former residents other than the public housing projects propelled the uprising of 1967. The raid of an unsanctioned bar that night in July was just the match in the powder barrel. The continued mass exodus of white residents to Detroit's suburbs (a 20 percent reduction in the city's population) and the auto industry's move abroad compounded the economic collapse, leaving many of the homes vacant and half the Black men unemployed by the time I was born.

After his stint in the army, my father's traceable work was as sporadic as his visits, which stopped altogether before I made it to middle school. Whenever my mother would learn of his employment, she threatened to pursue child support, and the next time we saw him, he'd be on to something else. He was the eldest son, but I never got the sense that he carried the weight of responsibility that came with having six younger siblings. I tried to piece together an image of him from the fragments he left behind—the scent of tobacco and cologne when he hugged me, a photograph of him and Magic Johnson in one of my mother's photo albums, how his easygoing manner seemed to linger in the air long after he was gone. But the pieces never quite fit together to paint much of a picture, leaving me with more questions than answers.

Surviving in this environment often meant accepting circumstances without harboring ambitions for more. Many men and women worked in factories facing obsolescence, rising before dawn for early shifts, their labor eclipsing the sunrise of a new day. For a high school graduate lacking specific trade skills in the 1980s, employment at Ford, General Motors, or Chrysler brought an average wage of nine to ten dollars an hour—three times the US minimum wage of three dollars and ten cents. I once asked Uncle Frank why he was always leaving for work as I was coming home from school and why he always complained of being tired. He lowered his head slightly, and responded, "There are a lot of men like me, and half of them need a job."

It would be easy to say that my dysfunctional home life was an inevitability, a byproduct of what was happening all around us. But I always managed to see it as both circumstantial and systemic. It was neither predetermined nor universal, even if deeply embedded. "The city of Detroit has been in financial difficulty for so long that it has become almost an article of faith that, somehow, it will manage," begins a 2013 article in *The Economist*. I remember reading it and immediately recalling the countless times we stood in long lines at Focus: HOPE to pick up powdered milk, canned fruit cocktail, and large orange bricks of "government cheese." I thought of the Christmases when we'd open our wrapped packages to find pairs of donated white tube socks and the Saturday afternoons when Leah and I would slide them on over our long johns before stepping into our snow suits and moon boots, dressed for hours of shoveling snow for elderly neighbors who'd kindly pay little girls five or six dollars for shoddy sidewalk clearing. Our history of "making a way out of no way" goes deeper than Detroit's financial woes and ensuing decline. This, too, was a way of living.

Tenacity born from scarcity may also become the catalyst for change. Under the pressure of scarcity, the brain can become skilled at swift decision-making, parsing choices with speed and precision, favoring those that promise immediate rewards. Honed by generations of hardship, the brain becomes expert at navigating the intricacies of scarcity, optimizing limited resources, and making do.

ॐ

When I last visited Detroit, I drove past the DIA on the way to my hotel. *The Thinker* once again beckoned to me, this time an invitation to reflect on the contrast between decay and renewal—how this city could be collapsing and flourishing at the same time. Driving through Detroit, I marvel at the way you can strategically sidestep ruin by confining yourself to certain neighborhoods. It is a calculated dance of avoidance, like dormant genes lying in wait. Abandoned factories bear the imprints of the automotive industry's rise and decline. Their skeletal remains stand as both monuments and warnings. The city's inner streets, once bustling and vivacious, lie as silent witnesses to the ebb and flow of life. I reckon with the glaring asymmetry of worth and value, while wishing for better things. I boomerang between hope and despair. But like a Detroiter, even one who left nearly thirty years ago, I hold faith in the city's future, however uncertain.

Faith that we were formed not in loyalty to the oppressive conditions around us, but in defiance of them. Each small act of survival, each creative solution to a seemingly insurmountable problem, is an assertion of our humanity and our right to exist fully, despite the constraints imposed upon us. Faith that this renewed spirit of transformation is equally contagious, a spark so powerful that it may ignite the lamps of the 634,000 people who stayed and have spent six decades waiting for the light.

5

REMNANTS OF A MOTHER

When you are not fed love on a silver
spoon, you learn to lick it off knives.

—Lauren Eden

If I asked my mother how old I was when she let me taste cocaine, I imagine her answer would be shrouded in the same haze that envelops many of our shared memories. Memories of a time marked by the erratic dance of her moods, the sharp contrast between euphoria and despair. But I was eight and it remains one of the few memories I have from that time that I remember with clarity. My mother, sister, and I were at her boyfriend Kenny's apartment, where cocaine was traded in Ziploc bags smaller than any I'd ever seen, and rocks sizzled beneath the flame of a cigarette lighter, cradled on a tarnished spoon. Kenny also worked at Chrysler, but I imagine it was the dealing that drew her to him. Being his girlfriend meant getting high whenever she wanted and without paying for it. Only when they smoked did we have to leave the room.

But when Kenny shook the cocaine out onto a plate and made lines with his driver's license, rolled up a dollar bill, and did a line, we were there for it all.

"Does it taste like sugar?" I asked, not yet aware of what it was.

My mother, nonchalant, wet the tip of her pinkie finger on her tongue, then dipped it in the residue. "Here," she offered, letting me lick it off her fingertip as if it were powdered sugar and she was baking a cake.

I knew from an early age that she wasn't like other moms. Women didn't usually welcome her presence around their husbands or boyfriends, and most kids in the neighborhood didn't venture beyond our front porch. We knew almost all of our neighbors by name, but there was no sense of community. Aside from the handful of times we were allowed to use someone's telephone to make an important phone call, most people kept to themselves. They'd speak when spoken to, but there were no neighborhood backyard barbecues or game nights. I believe Mama had borrowed money from many of them at one point or another. I imagine she still owes them to this day. I never knew her to have real girlfriends. There had been her grade school friend, Tammy, whom at one point she called our "godmother," but I only remember seeing her a handful of times. Mama's relationships, where they existed, were transactional and, usually, with men. The people she spent time with weren't friends so much as associates in a network of scavengers who agreed to smoke whatever any of them could come up with. My understanding of her difference metastasized into the idea that I might inherit this same distinctiveness, and that my survival depended on guarding against anything resembling her kind of different.

I often allowed her the illusion that she was hiding her truth from me. Our relationship hinged on this unspoken understanding. A dance of knowing without acknowledging, of witnessing without intervening. I became skilled at navigating the spaces between her words, of deciphering the unsaid, of concealing the truths I stumbled upon, sharing them only with Leah if at all. Those basement nights, the comings and goings, the silences and sounds, painted a tableau of my mother's struggles. A world she never intended for me to see, but that, despite her efforts, became the backdrop of our shared existence.

I rationalized that if Mama was okay, I would be too. But she wasn't okay. I rode the drift of her moods, learning to recognize the warning signs of an impending storm or the deceptive calm. Her restlessness manifested in chain-smoking and obsessive cleaning, activities that seemed to offer her hands a purpose. Everything in the house smelled of Newport cigarettes, but you could eat off the kitchen floor.

Mama often sent us to the store to keep her stash in stock. The quarter-mile walk to Sam's Party Shoppe was mostly on our street, but it was a long block that curved out of view before turning onto Chicago Road. The first time I walked there alone, I felt uneasy about who I might encounter. Two men loitered along the way, their faces obscured by my peripheral vision. Each step closer to them felt like walking into an unknown threat. They didn't look like they wanted to hurt me, but they didn't look like they wouldn't. I kept my gaze fixed ahead, my steps quickening, my heart in my ears.

As I reached the first crosswalk, I met the familiar, sweet smell of Bays English muffins being made in the factory across the street. Inside Sam's, the fluorescent lights buzzed overhead, and the scent of English muffins morphed into malt liquor and potato chips. I pushed past the arcade games that we'd play once tall enough to reach them. I could barely see over the counter, but I immediately spotted my target—the row of plastic containers of Starburst, Nerds, Red Hots, Lemon Heads, and flavored Tootsie Rolls—and made eye contact with Sam, who watched a small TV behind bulletproof plexiglass. As he approached, I placed a purple one-dollar food stamp onto the counter.

"Can I have two cherry Tootsie Rolls and two pink Starburst, please?" I asked, sliding the food stamp toward the small opening for cash. They were five cents each, which meant I could buy eight loosies with the change.

We couldn't buy cigarettes with food stamps, but if we bought candy with the one-dollar food stamp, we'd get cash back and use the change to buy Mama's cigarettes. If Leah and I went together, we could get her a pack. We had done it dozens of times, but I always felt a rumble in my stomach, as if we were doing something wrong and at risk of getting into trouble.

Sam set the candy down, then counted out the change on the counter before sliding it all through the open slot. I counted the change again, as I'd been taught to do, before placing it back in the slot for the cigarettes, which Sam tucked into a small brown paper bag. I appreciated his discretion, which, in hindsight, was likely more about protecting himself than honoring my sense of privacy.

Then there were the euphoric first few days of each month when she received her welfare payment consisting of some three hundred dollars in food stamps and a check for two hundred and twenty dollars, which I remember being just enough for the monthly mortgage payment on our side of the duplex. When she was flush, grocery shopping day was better than Christmas. We would go on a big food shopping spree, my mother filling the grocery cart with things we could manage without her: boxes of cereal, cans of Chef Boyardee ravioli, hot dogs and lunch meat, Wonder Bread, peanut butter. She also bought eggs and bacon or sausage that she'd sometimes cook for us on late weekend mornings, and canned salmon, which she loved to fry into patties with diced onions, or fried chicken that she served with frozen broccoli or canned creamed corn. But whatever we procured on that one trip usually had to last the entire month because she would trade the remaining food stamps for cash, never at a one-to-one ratio.

One afternoon, I was so hungry that I decided to go food shopping myself. I rode my bike about a mile from home to the nearest grocery store to get enough for the week. I carried a small duffel bag that I wore cross-body and took everything from packages of sausage links and ham to Pop-Tarts and small cans of fruit cocktail. Milk was too heavy, and bread took up too much space. I can only imagine now how obvious I must have been. I remember being self-conscious about being there alone, but no one said anything to me. I was nine or so and it was the 1980s, a time when six-year-olds learned how to tell analog time and knew the walking route home from school. By the time I was six, I also had a set of house keys and had taught Leah how to tie her shoes.

I filled the duffel with as much as I could and made it out of the store. As I rode my bike home, the bag knocked against my leg, slowing me down. I felt shame for what I had done, but I also felt victorious. I had accomplished something meaningful, and was high from the rush of competence and pride in knowing that we would have food at the house. The second time, I got caught, and the man threatened to call the police. I never shoplifted again.

Instead, we made a habit of collecting empty soda cans and bottles for the nickel or dime deposits we'd get for their return. We rarely had enough for an impressive haul, so Mama would make us ask Uncle Frank or a couple of neighbors if they had any that we could have. It's a wonder I survived the shame of having to knock on doors to ask and then of having to carry thirty-gallon trash bags full of them to the store.

And then there was the wild look in her eyes, one I came to know well. It was as if the very essence of my mother had been replaced by something alien, desperate. The restlessness became focused, a heat-seeking missile that dismantled the house, targeting money or anything valuable enough to sell. If she discovered that a family member or friend had gifted us five or ten dollars for birthdays or meals, she'd ransack our bedroom, overturning mattresses, rifling through drawers, violating any box or nook where I stashed my "precious" belongings—a journal, a piece of costume jewelry from a Christmas when my paternal grandmother felt generous.

If we were at school during such a fit, Leah and I would come home to find that the TV, VCR, or microwave had also mysteriously "vanished." We eventually pieced together that she was selling them for cash. After a few months, she'd somehow replace them—either with part of her monthly welfare payment or through the generosity of a man smitten with her, only for her to sell the replacements a few months later.

She'd then leave, seeking the promise that she would be able to live within her own mind. Sometimes for the day, sometimes overnight, gradually extending into more prolonged absences. By the time I was thirteen, she could be gone for two to three days at a time. As scary as it was for her to leave, unsure of when she'd return, it was petrifying to accompany her because that meant waiting outside in the car for hours. I'd sit in the front seat like I was protecting the car, while deathly afraid that someone would come take the car and me along with it. It was during those lonely dark hours that I would listen to the radio and dream of the life I'd someday have. More than once, I spent the night sleeping in that car, awaking with the sunrise.

But the rage? It was like trying to contain the ocean. On more occasions than I can recall, I found my mother, hollow-eyed and red-nosed, fighting in the street with the neighbor over trivialities that no longer mattered by the end of their disputes. There would be foot chases in bare feet and hair pulling, swinging fists until someone fell to the ground, usually bringing the street theater to an end. Mama was quick to curse or swing in anger, and eventually it ceased to matter what had sparked her initial fury; in the aftermath, you were still a "low-down dirty motherfucker," her words sharp enough to slice through the thickest of skins. Depending on the nature of the offense, *dirty* might be swapped for a different adjective. Leah and I risked being labeled *selfish* if we inadvertently provoked her by consuming the last bit of food at home, in which case we might also be *greedy*. She had a penchant for *stupid*, *ugly*, and *slutty*, all readily accessible, particularly when coming down from her high and grappling with the frustration of inadequate funds for her next fix. The very essence of her being was held captive by a force that transcended conscious control.

And then there were the downtimes, as I'd come to understand them—stretches of profound melancholy that left her confined to bed for days. When she descended into that subterranean world, it was as if a curtain fell, hiding her from herself and the world. She never seemed to find that line between smoothing out the edges versus tapping out completely.

Only later, when I began to learn about the neuroscience of addiction, did I find some understanding in the words of Dr. Gabor Maté, renowned addiction expert. After decades of treating people with substance abuse problems, his compassion and his wisdom made me rethink much of what I thought I knew about her struggle. "It is impossible to understand addiction without asking what relief the addict finds, or hopes to find, in the drug or the addictive behaviour," he offers. "The question is not why the addiction, but why the pain." Only in recent years have I been able to reflect on and appreciate the heart of this inquiry, as I grappled with the realization that her struggle was not merely a battle against external circumstances. It was against a far deeper hurt, one rooted in both her body and her past, shaped by a complex dance of genetics and environment.

It's been said that pain travels through families until someone is ready to feel it. The cycle of addiction, of pain, had been passed down like an heirloom. Her descent into those dark spaces was a continuation of a larger, intergenerational narrative.

I told myself that my mother's undoing happened suddenly, like the car accident that claimed Grandma's life. But her unraveling was most certainly gradual, a process that likely started when she was just twelve. Home alone with Grandpa Billy one day, she discovered him lifeless. One version of the story says that he died of a brain tumor. The other is that he took his own life.

"He blew his brains out, and I found him dead," she would say, sparing the details of the gunshot and its aftermath.

Grandpa's suicide, an unspeakable tragedy, was etched into our family history, a shadowy legacy that left me with unanswered questions. Mama had been the only person to ever speak of it, usually as a plea for sympathy. The details of Grandpa's past were sparse—half-remembered facts about a man born to a Native mother and white father in Arkansas, one of thirteen children, a Navy veteran with a drinking problem and a brain tumor. Whatever inner battles he fought, they were buried with him, leaving behind only the pain he passed on.

I used to wonder how that day shaped her—how finding him like that had marked her, how it had twisted her relationship with Grandma. Did it draw them closer, or did it fracture them too? One more story buried in the depths of silence. All that remained of him was his naval portrait, which sat prominently in our living room; his piercing blue eyes and easy smile made me long to know him too.

As a result, I don't know much else about my maternal grandparents' life together. They were both married and each had children before finding each other. They were born just one day apart—his birthday was Valentine's Day, hers the day before—an almost poetic symmetry of their union. Grandma brought three sons to the marriage—all of whom she'd had by age twenty—and Grandpa Billy had two sons with his first wife. Grandma and Grandpa were both twenty-seven when my mother was born.

As the youngest and the only daughter, Mama grew up intelligent and spoiled. I watched her find men to take care of her, witnessing many unfamiliar faces, shadows that crept in during the darkest hours, their exchanges cloaked in secrecy. Our home was a revolving door for the many men in her life—young and old, clean and addicted—none of them able to resist her hazel doe eyes and wide smile, or her high, rounded cheekbones, and sandy brown wavy hair. She was born a blonde, a fact in which she took great pride, and she stood more than five feet seven inches tall. And none of them, not even the most discerning among them, were a match for her beauty and cunning. Mama showed me how even the smartest man was stupid when it came to a woman he wanted. When she was high, even her beauty became blurred, a constellation of freckles punctuated by the deepest of dimples, one in each cheek. Still, she recognized the power in her beauty, and she valued it highly, never hesitating to use it to get what she wanted or needed.

Among her more enduring "relationships" was with Patrick Rome, a divorced electrician with two children and a penchant for beer and brown liquor. His beady eyes were often bloodshot, and he stood with a posture that apologized for his existence. While not conventionally attractive, Patrick compensated with a disarming, albeit pitiful, self-deprecating humor and an unparalleled generosity. Despite hailing from some level of affluence, he maintained a distant relationship with his family, a likely consequence of an underlying mental disorder and barely functioning alcoholism.

Patrick was obsessed with my mother. I'd seen many men come and go in her life, but few of them worshipped her the way he did. He did so with an intensity that made me somewhat afraid of him. He seemed to want to possess her in a way that felt inhuman, like she was a trophy or a pet. And from what I could tell, his devotion knew no bounds; he would do anything for her, legal or otherwise. Most often, this included jeopardizing his electrician's license by illegally reconnecting our power, disregarding the escalating notices from Detroit Edison—green, yellow, and finally, pink.

One night around 2 a.m., Patrick came seeking solace from my mother. But she refused him. First, he begged her to let him in. She continued to refuse him entry, which set off a cacophony of screams that woke us. Leah and I went downstairs to find them yelling at each other through the side door.

"Don't play with me, Carolyn. I will cut your fucking lights off!" he threatened.

"Do what you want, you ain't getting in!" she screamed back at him.

Patrick grew silent and within minutes, we had no power. His threat wasn't idle.

"Carolyn, let me in. I just want to talk. I need to talk to you. Then I'll turn the lights back on."

Mama continued to scream at him as he yelled now from the back of the house where he'd disconnected the electricity. Impatience fueling his anger, Patrick shattered one of the kitchen windows, despite the security bars covering the exterior of every window. He broke the window to piss her off and to make a point. It wasn't the first broken window our house suffered, and it wouldn't be the last, but it was the most frightening. Furious at his audacity, she began coaxing him to the side door, promising to talk to him and maybe even let him in. By then, Leah and I were wide-awake, fearfully standing guard.

"I'll show his ass," she declared, a forewarning of the impending reckoning.

Drawing inspiration from the infamous incident involving Al Green's girlfriend years before, my mother swiftly brought a can of old bacon grease to a crackling boil. She lured Brian back to the door and threw it on him, covering his face and eventually his hands, with which he reflexively shielded his burning skin. I was in such shock that I didn't initially feel the hot grease that splattered back onto me, scorching my hands and right arm, leaving blistered reminders that lasted for weeks.

My mother was not without kindness. When she was up, she told me how smart I was, how proud of me she was. It made me believe I could save her with my goodness, but there was no smile or sacrifice big enough to meet her needs. It didn't take much for her to turn on me, ignore me, berate me, or accuse me of terrible things. She knew what hurt and she struck hard and to the core. Whatever love that was there was overshadowed by an inability to forgive our mere existence. Someone must pay for life's injustices, after all, and my father was out of reach.

Even in her sober moments, the mantle of motherhood seemed difficult for her, and the struggle was etched on her sleeve, a tattoo on her wrist that stayed in my constant line of sight. Leah and I kept growing while everything seemed to shrink. And as our needs increased, Mama had less to give. She never really earned a living; when she worked, the month-long stints at Rite Aid or the grocery store always ended abruptly. Motherhood felt like one of the many jobs she abandoned. I felt like an adversary to her addiction, drafted into a war I had no chance of winning. The unconditional love I longed for remained elusive, and the desire for it lingered, the want of which I feared I would never escape.

I know there were good times, good feelings, good memories. I look for them sometimes. When I think of my mother, though, there's mostly just a collection of painful remembrances, experiences that would later seem incomprehensible, like the night she came home with a black eye and a bloody gash on her head after someone pistol-whipped her. She said that she had been robbed but it seems far more likely that either she'd stolen from someone or she owed them money.

I often wondered, though never dared to ask, why she didn't just give us up when we were young. Why not entrust our care to our grandparents or explore adoption? I suspect she sentimentalized motherhood too much, having lost her own. Letting us go might have felt like conceding defeat. She was willing to falter in her role as a mother; she simply couldn't bring herself to admit the failure. She did eventually decide that raising us was an unbearable burden, but by then, Leah and I were in high school, and I had grown tired of asking questions that went unanswered. I hadn't realized people gave up fourteen- and fifteen-year-olds. We weren't kicked out for bad behavior. We hadn't threatened to run away. We were dropped off like unwanted extras in the litter. One evening we were simply told to pack a few belongings because we were going away for a while. I tried to glean something from her expression, but her face was a closed book, her gaze already drifting to some point beyond us. And with a faraway look in her eyes she told us that we were going to stay with her aunt Claudia. She didn't say why or for how long.

I left my childhood home not knowing that it would be forever.

For six or seven months, we lived with Aunt Claudia with no sense of where our mother had gone. After failed efforts to locate her, we found my dad and all but made him take us in. He lived, respectfully, in a shithole. Aside from mattresses in the two bedrooms, and a small table with two chairs in the kitchen, there was very little furniture. We went from never having spent the night with him to living with him for the first time in our lives. I was surprised that he even agreed to take us in.

It wasn't long before he began complaining about all of the driving he suddenly had to do with us around and asking me for gas money. We lasted two months there, finishing the school year before acknowledging that we were worse off with him. At least the house we grew up in with Mama was ours. Our stuff was there, and it was safer to walk down the street. After the school year ended, we moved in with Aunt Rochelle, one of my father's best friend's sisters. To this day, I have no idea what anyone said for her to agree to let two teenagers she barely knew stay with her, but she took us in for the summer. We babysat her five-year-old daughter while she worked, a reasonable way to pay for her generous hospitality.

Leah remained relentless in her search for our mother

though, and one day, she found her. She learned that Mama was living with an old man she had met at some point during our estrangement—Mr. Charles—in his house on the east side of Detroit.

"I want to go be with Mama," Leah insisted.

"But it's not even her place; she's living with some man," I reasoned. "We don't even know if there's room for us." As angry as I had been with her for leaving us at Aunt Claudia's, I also wanted to see her. I just wasn't sure I could handle it if she didn't really want us back.

"I know, but I'd rather be with her than stay here. She talked to him about it and said we could come."

We debated our scant options and agreed to leave Aunt Rochelle's to be with Mama at Mr. Charles's house. Leah didn't want to be without our mother, and I didn't want to be without Leah. We packed up what little we had and moved into the shoddy two-bedroom house on Wexford Street, where we stayed through my entire junior year and the start of senior year of high school. Leah moved into the spare bedroom with Mama, and I found a corner in the living room to make "mine," sleeping on the twenty-some-year-old plastic-wrapped sofa. It was so old that the plastic had turned a brownish yellow, matching the sofa it shielded. On the floor to the right of the sofa, I kept my clothes in neat piles. On the left sat the boombox I begged my mother to buy me as a middle school graduation present.

Despite the condition of the house, it felt nice to be

reunited. Mom looked pretty good. She had gained some weight, a sign that she had an appetite and was perhaps actually doing well. Mr. Charles was in his late sixties, maybe early seventies, and my mother had taken the ironic role of his caregiver and live-in companion. Usually, the men in her life moved in with us—Daniel, Tim, then Eric. I didn't fully understand the nature of their relationship, but they seemed content to have each other. That August, I got a job working at Express at Eastland Mall, so between work, cheer practice, and dance rehearsals, I spent as much time out of the house as possible. We enjoyed this new normal for the rest of the summer, but it didn't take long for her old behavior of sneaking around, staying out overnight, and spending her days home in bed to resurface.

She was still using.

6

HOUSE OF CARDS

My mother, the person who should have been my sanctuary, was often my greatest source of fear. Safety and security were illusions. I had to learn to be vigilant, to tread cautiously through always uncertain terrain. This constant sense of instability at home shaped the way I would learn to interact with the outside world, which I did not view as a safe place. My solution was to forge a path defined by the relentless pursuit of control.

I focused on school, which was orderly and predictable. I ensured that I looked the part. Even as my clothes began to look worn, I kept them clean and pressed. I learned to wash and iron them, putting creases in my pants the way I'd seen my teachers wear. And most importantly, I kept my vow of silence, believing my secrets kept me safe. But a closer look would show the many manifestations of secret keeping well into my adulthood. Even if we think we've disconnected from them, the memories and feelings that accompany the most harrowing events of our lives get lodged in our brains and our bodies. I hadn't clocked the nerves bad enough to foster a nail-biting habit until I was twenty-five, when I also learned that my jaw was perpetually clenched, the muscles so taut that a dentist called it to my attention. He asked if I suffered from headaches or pain while chewing. I had no such afflictions and couldn't understand why he was asking.

"You have some of the most developed jaw muscles I've ever seen. If there was such a thing as bodybuilding facial muscles, you'd be a fierce competitor," he joked. "A lot of people clench when they're stressed."

Stressed. I had swallowed every slight, slap, and snarl, until they became lodged deep in a place beyond language. My stomach became the repository for my pain. As a child and young adult, I had a very difficult time having bowel movements. I blamed it on a scavenger's diet of processed foods. But I'd never known how it felt to have a stomach free from knots. It was always knotted—from hunger or from fear—and I couldn't let it out.

Every evening my mother failed to come back home left me nauseous. I vomited the night she did return, with a black eye after someone hit her. I prayed that the chocolate milk in my free lunch would soothe the sour stomach that accompanied me to school the mornings after someone threw a brick through the front living room window. At sixteen, I'd be rushed to the emergency room for an ulcer the doctor said was "due to stress." The pain of being my mother's daughter was eating me alive.

As I began to navigate the landscape of my own cravings as an adult, my awareness turned to the tightrope I often walked between filling my stomach and feeding a deprivation that transcended my physical appetite. Eating, for me, had become an attempt to quiet the hunger that lived within me. I ate to nourish a hunger for love, for my significance. Being full was an affirmation—a way to anchor myself in a world that felt untethered. Fill myself to feel the weight of my existence, the reassurance of gravity, a tangible proof that I am cared for because my belly is full, that my presence is acknowledged through the simple, necessary act of being nourished.

But there's a fine line between satisfying hunger and drowning in excess. I constantly pushed those boundaries, attempting to fill a void that doesn't yield to the comfort of food. Intent on feeling my weight, evidence that I'm not a ghost, I wanted to believe that this fullness would bring a sense of completeness, that in the moment, I would feel like I am enough. Needing oxytocin but settling for dopamine. As the nausea sets in, I recognize the sick feeling is not just a physical response; it's a visceral acknowledgment that I have tried to address a longing that cannot be satiated. I am full, but I am not enough.

For girls without mothers or maternal figures suffer an injury that author and licensed professional counselor Kelly

McDaniel calls mother hunger, the feeling of terminal brokenness, of primal fear of abandonment, or disordered boundaries, a wound that resides deep within the right brain as a result of not receiving adequate nurturance, protection, and guidance in the early years of maternal attachment.

The right hemisphere of the brain is associated with emotions, creativity, and nonverbal communication, making it a crucial center for processing and interpreting the emotional landscape. A right brain wound, in this context, might manifest as an impaired ability to regulate emotions effectively. The emotional neglect from a disinterested mother can result in difficulties recognizing, expressing, or understanding one's own emotions. There may be a heightened vulnerability to emotional overwhelm, as the typical regulatory mechanisms are compromised. The right hemisphere is also integral to the development of interpersonal connections and our ability to attune to others emotionally. Absent or disinterested parents may contribute to challenges in forming healthy relationships, characterized by difficulties in understanding and responding to emotional cues in oneself or others.

In my case, my self-image had been all but shattered. A kind of dysmorphia, like staring at a word for so long that it no longer looks right. The spelling suddenly seems off. The emotional neglect I suffered left me feeling insecure, unworthy, and with a persistent sense of needing validation of my place in the world. Pleasing, perfecting, and performing at the highest levels became cornerstones of my identity at a very young age, survival tools that I would wield masterfully throughout my childhood and rely on into my thirties. This armor guaranteed my safety, and it won me praise, acceptance, scholarships, and, ultimately, a way out.

It also kept me disconnected.

Growing up, I didn't have a best friend. It was too risky an endeavor, a luxury I couldn't afford. A best friend—my best friend—would have come over for playdates and sleepovers. She might have noticed the lack of food in our house; that our utilities were routinely turned off, leaving us without heat, electricity, running water, or a working telephone; that strangers came and went at all hours; and that my mother often didn't come home at all. A friend might ask questions or mention these curiosities to her parents, who would in turn call Child Protective Services—an entity whose name I knew and feared from a very young age. My mother often dangled CPS as a threat, saying that if anyone "told," Leah and I would be taken away and placed separately in foster homes, a fate far worse than life with her.

"If you think you'll have it better somewhere else, go find out," she'd say. "First of all, no one will want you. And if they take you, they won't take you both. You'll be split up. And if there's a man in the house, he'll probably rape you. So, call them if you want."

The routine deprivations of electricity, gas, running water, and a working telephone became grim constants of our lives. Rarely did we have more than two at once, and I can barely remember a time when we had them all functioning at the same time. No matter how cold the house got or how bored we were without television, or even how embarrassing it was not to have a working telephone (I stopped giving my phone number to friends at school when I realized it could lead to the shame of a classmate saying, "I tried to call you, but it said your phone was disconnected"), nothing was worse than having our water shut off.

On two different occasions that I can remember, for months at a time, we had no running water at home. This meant that at least six times a day, Leah and I had to fill pails of water from a neighbor's hose and carry them across the driveways and up the side steps back to the house. Using this water to cook or so that we could flush the toilet was relatively easy. Bathing was an altogether different logistical challenge. To take a "bath," we had to heat up large pots of water on the stove, or hot plate when the gas was off, then mix the scalding hot water with cool water to get the right temperature for washing up. We got the recipe for the bathing water down to a science: one part boiling water to two and a half parts cold water.

It was impossible to get enough water for a real bath. That would have taken too long and far too many trips up and down the stairs. Instead, we'd bathe directly out of the half-full five-gallon paint buckets that we used for fetching the water from our neighbor's outdoor faucet and that Uncle

Frank otherwise used for fishing. The pails stayed stacked up by the side door, and whenever one of us needed to take a bath, or do laundry on the washboard, we'd grab two and go out and around to Uncle Frank's side or head ten feet across the driveways to sneak water from the spigot on the side of our next-door neighbor Mrs. Fears's house. Needless to say, I stayed as clean as I possibly could. Mama's bath time was always the most inconvenient—when we were out playing in the yard with the boys in our neighborhood.

"DariaLeah! I need some water! One of you go get it."

We agreed to take turns, so whoever did it most recently would look at the other and say, "Your turn!"

We always tried to be discreet, but our friends must have had some sense of what we were doing. If they did, they never uttered a word.

Michigan winters, unforgiving and harsh, were especially difficult. So, when the gas had been turned off, we had to warm our room with a broken space heater with no protective vent, just two poles that burned bright red when hot. If we had gas but no electricity, the oven became a makeshift fireplace. We would preheat it and once it reached the target temperature, we opened the oven door and let all the heat into the house. (It never ceased to astound me how many shut-off warnings utilities companies would send when you didn't pay your bills. I would spend weeks in anticipation of losing running water or electricity or gas heating.) My mother kept the kerosene heater downstairs and a nicer space heater to herself—the one she used with her "friends" during their retreats to the basement. I shivered constantly and sometimes, I'd swear I could see my breath in the house. I slept in layered long sleeves and pants, tucked into my acrylic Barbie sleeping bag. One night, I fell asleep with the space heater too close to my bed and was suddenly awakened by the smell and heat of the sleeping bag burning, melting right in front of my eyes. Luckily there was no real fire. I shook the sleeping bag until I was able to beat out the small flame before it spread. And although it bore the unbearable smell of burnt plastic and the singed edge curled into a hard crust, I slept in it for years.

To survive meant blurring the lines between fantasy and reality, between the child I was and the self-made parent I had to become. It was a struggle that defined my life for many years, the delicate interplay between appearing as a child and wearing the armor of an adult. The intimate details of my family dysfunction remained carefully held secrets while I adopted the mantle of a self-appointed guardian, crafting the facade of a girl who was well cared for—a generous smile, pristine clothes, perfect grades, and my absolute best behavior in school. Being an A student meant no requests for parent-teacher meetings. When they occurred, they were solo endeavors, where I often found myself, a fifth grader, coming up with new excuses for the irregularities in my attendance. *What would I say this time?* One can be *that* sick only so many times.

Today, in the Detroit Public School system, students who

have missed at least 10 percent of the school year are considered chronically absent. I couldn't tell you what the policy was in the late '80s and early '90s, but there were a few years when we missed far more than that. I remember several instances when we dodged DPS truancy officers who came to the house to investigate. On other occasions, my paternal grandmother fielded calls from the school and drove over to our house herself. Sometimes, we talked to her through the door. If permitted inside, she seldom ventured beyond the threshold, inquiring why we weren't in school and where my mother was. Upon learning that she was upstairs "asleep," she'd raise her voice.

"Carolyn? The school called again trying to reach you. These kids need to be in school. I'm not going to keep making excuses for you. Next time, I'm going to let them come over here themselves. Carolyn, I know you hear me."

There would be stretches—sometimes as long as two weeks—when my mother kept us home from school. Mornings meant to offer a routine, a structured escape from the chaos of my home life, were instead disrupted by my mother's desperate longing for company and care after a night out. My routine was set: I would prepare my folders and notebooks and pick my clothes for school the night before, mimicking what I had seen my mother do for us in earlier years. Yet, more often than not, my mother's return with the sunrise, erratic behavior, and insatiable need for companionship derailed my hopes for finding refuge at school.

"Stay with me today," Mom would implore from behind the alien eyes where she kept herself.

"I haven't been to school in over a week," I would appeal.

To appear wounded, she'd pout, adding, "I need you. Just one more day."

As much as I hated missing school and dreaded the day I'd go back after being out for weeks, I feared denying her while sometimes relishing in the idea that my presence offered her solace.

Walking those four and a half blocks to school filled me with great anxiety. My stomach churned as I sifted through excuses for my extended absence... Had someone died last time? Maybe my mother was sick. Or I was. On the playground or in the lunch line, waves of paranoia would swell in me, and I'd suddenly wonder if they could all tell, if I was the subject of their private amusement. Like going on about my day with something in my teeth or toilet paper stuck to my shoe. Did neglected children exude a particular smell? Were we missing the sweet scent of nurture, perceptible to everyone around us?

Having been promoted early to first grade—before my fifth birthday—I began middle school at nine years old. The truancy continued, and at the end of that school year, I was held back, forced to repeat the sixth grade. I was mortified. School had been my sanctuary and the nucleus of my self-esteem. There, I was validated, recognized by teachers for my intelligence and diligence. In textbooks and lesson plans, the world made sense. I happily took on the extra-credit assignments. The classroom was a stage where I could perform, and my academic achievements were the applause that could drown out the storm that raged at home. Each high mark on a test or a well-deserved commendation fueled my sense of self-worth, which was under constant assault at home.

In the tender spaces where validation should have grown, the seeds of my self-esteem struggled to take root. My hard work to prove that I mattered was no longer fortified. This failure showed me that the foundation I'd attempted to build was flimsy. I was losing the plot: Get an education and get out. I felt my dreams slipping away and it terrified me. I also felt great shame but refused anything resembling self-pity. Though intimately familiar with it herself, my mother regarded self-pity as the worst of traits in others. My tears were often met with her anger. It was unacceptable for her to have a weak and sensitive child. I adopted this sentiment, a shield I would wield against even my most vulnerable moments.

In the language of therapy, my approach to survival would be described as an adaptive coping mechanism. Early in my childhood, I sculpted my identity and crafted responses to my world in pursuit of a comforting sense of safety. In making these decisions, some of which I made unconsciously while others were made with eyes wide open, I embraced certain qualities while purposefully severing ties with others. Opting for approval meant warding off the prospect of disappointing people. When my early life was threatening, I cocooned myself within a protective emotional shell, burying anything that might be used against me. The guiding principle was crystal clear: The better I became at adapting, the more practiced I grew in excising conflicting thoughts, feelings, and traits that threatened to lead me astray.

Failing sixth grade was a wake-up call. My ten-year-old rock bottom. The determination I had to get away from my life intensified, fueled by the fear of being trapped in that cycle of dysfunction and poverty. In my case, the absence of maternal nurturing birthed in me a drive to succeed. I completed sixth and seventh grade at the same school, and in deep shame. I decided that I would not spend another school year with my failure hanging over me. I made my mom transfer me to a new school before eighth grade, and I started over. I would have to take the bus to school because it wasn't in our neighborhood, but I didn't care. I didn't know anyone there and could reinvent myself. I tried out for and joined the cheer team and sharpened my laser focus on my escape plan.

I first learned about Renaissance from Mrs. Slater, my eighth-grade geometry teacher, who also coached our competitive cheer team. Mrs. Slater was in her early thirties and was the coolest adult I knew. She was young enough to know and like a lot of the music we were into, but she had the maturity and experience to command the deep respect of a classroom of thirteen- and fourteen-year-olds. She was the kind of adult you wanted to impress. One afternoon before cheer practice, a few months before the entrance exam, Mrs. Slater presumptively asked the eighth-grade girls on the squad which high schools we were applying to. Two of the girls mentioned plans to attend their neighborhood high school. She squinted at them with feigned confusion, a look that said she thought what they were saying was ridiculous. Two other girls each named their top choice. That made her smile. I had heard murmurs about the application process at that point but knew nothing about any of the schools. When she got to me, I said, "I'm not sure. I need to do more research." I got a nod of satisfaction. (In my experience, "Let me look into it and get back to you" is a foolproof response.)

After practice, I asked Mrs. Slater which was the best of the three and if she thought one would be ideal for me.

"Cass Tech is the oldest and the biggest. They have about three thousand students. It's all the way downtown, but it's a great school. Students have a mix of college prep and technical course work. Diana Ross went there." *Interesting data point. She left and thrived.*

Three thousand kids, though? Hard pass. I think all I could manage was "Oh wow."

"Renaissance is the newest and the smallest and, therefore, the most competitive. There are only a couple hundred students in each class, and they have the best reputation for college prep. And it's here on the west side." *This Renaissance was generative.*

"That sounds perfect for me. I'm going to Renaissance then." In my mind, it was settled. I didn't even pretend that I'd need to discuss it with my mom, and I didn't bother to ask Mrs. Slater about the third school.

At Renaissance, I met upper-middle-class Black people for the first time. They were rich as far as I was concerned. Their parents were dentists, lawyers, professors, and businesspeople. They had degrees and credentials. One girl's mother was a judge. They went on family vacations and lived in neighborhoods with names. They belonged to organizations like Jack and Jill and were expected to pledge the same sorority or fraternity as their parents. As part of the Detroit Public School System, Renaissance was still predominantly Black, although it was more ethnically and socioeconomically diverse than the other public schools in the city. The curriculum attracted students from all over Detroit, and as Mrs. Slater promised, there were only two hundred or so kids in my incoming class. Many of my classmates lived in the most affluent, historic neighborhoods of Palmer Woods, Indian Village, and the Boston-Edison District—enclaves that largely went unscathed as other neighborhoods fell to ruin. These homes had originally been built for prominent Detroiters of the late nineteenth and early twentieth centuries, and their driveways held a car for every person of driving age in the home. For us, neighborhood status was determined less by proximity to whiteness, as was often the case in other inner cities, and more by the size of your home and the number of influential people you called "neighbor."

For the first time in my life, I was immersed in a river where we were all swimming in the same direction. To be smart was table stakes. Competence was ordinary. Success was expected. College was a given. Most of us were certified nerds, but it was cool to care. My pursuit of excellence felt like more than perfectionism. It was a function of my belief in an ideal world. In that, I found belonging. I auditioned for and joined the cheer team and the school's dance company, although I had never studied dance before my freshman modern dance class. I found outlets and became a part of teams, a bit of stability even as I moved six times between sophomore and senior year, living in seven different homes during those four years, one of which where my mother was absent from my life. Still, I clutched my secrets, pressed them between praying hands that pleaded for admission into an esteemed university and for graduation day to come without anyone finding out.

Renaissance, with its expectations and communal drive for success, became a cradle for my ambitions. The sense of community, the shared standard of excellence, the consistent and unwavering support of my teachers and, for the first time, real friends, created a powerful force that propelled me. I felt my dreams solidify into plans, my hopes into certainties. There I learned the true power of being immersed in a nurturing environment, one that could acknowledge the harsh realities of life while cultivating the spirit to rise above them. Some people had been made in Detroit's image, and some of us were formed not in loyalty to the conditions around us, but in defiance of them. Renaissance embodied that defiance. It was more than a school; it was a proving ground for the kind of tenacity that brought dreams to life. And I was not just a student; I was part of a movement to demonstrate the strength that comes from community, the possibility that arises from shared vision, and the undeniable truth that even in the midst of scarcity, we can create spaces of abundance and hope.

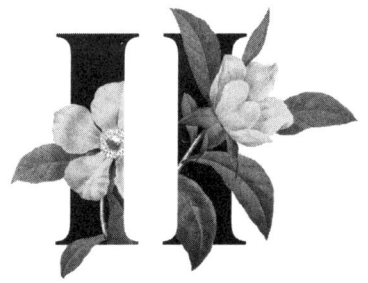

RECKONING

Your vision will become clear only when you can look into your own heart. Who looks outside, dreams; who looks inside, awakens.

—Carl Jung

7

EXODUS

The day I left for Ann Arbor felt like stepping into the sun after a long, dark night. As the last item was loaded into the trunk of Leah's boyfriend Samuel's car, I bade a silent farewell to the remains of my childhood. My spirit had somehow survived, and I clutched my newfound freedom, fleeing with it like a fugitive in the night. The drive to my dorm would take less than an hour, but it was a world away from Detroit.

At the University of Michigan, I immediately got involved in dance and theater. I felt like the best version of myself onstage. By the end of my first semester of freshman year I had already auditioned for and performed in the first of four university musicals and student-produced plays (two of which were crafted by Tony-nominated playwright Dominique Morisseau). Having become friends with Dominique and two other juniors—Maisha and Karma—who were also in the play, I was invited to join them on a spring break trip to the Bahamas. The destination was Nassau, where they had planned to stay for the week under the hospitality of Maisha's aunt and uncle. We would all have to share a room, but I thought they were the absolute coolest women I'd ever met, and I had never gone on such a vacation before, let alone to a Caribbean island for a beach getaway in the middle of winter. I was going to have the kind of college spring break that I had seen on TV. I got my very first credit card to fund the flight and acquire a few essentials in preparation for the trip. This was a moment.

Stepping off the plane in Nassau felt like walking onto a meticulously crafted movie set. Even the airport had a vibe, a fusion of tropical warmth and the rhythmic beats of reggae. As we emerged into the Bahamian sunlight, the air embraced us with a gentle caress, carrying the sweet scent of saltwater and blooming bougainvillea. Palm trees swayed lazily against the backdrop of an azure sky, their fronds rustling secrets only the island knew. The vibrant hues of the landscape painted a vivid contrast to the monotony of Michigan winter. It was a bit of sensory overload at times, but my senses drank deeply from the intoxicating essence of this new world. The Bahamian air, infused with the spirit of freedom and adventure, signaled the beginning of this new chapter in my life.

Our mornings unfolded around the dining table, where we enjoyed fresh fruit while we planned the day's escapades.

Maisha's cousin, a male companion our age with a vibrant social life in Nassau, happily assumed the role of tour guide to four American girls from Detroit. After breakfast, we'd visit one beach or another for a few hours, then walk around town to do a bit of sightseeing and souvenir hunting, usually returning home for dinner before venturing out for the night. On two occasions, her cousin took us to Paradise Island, where we got to spend the day at the newly named Atlantis Paradise Island as guests of his friend who worked there. Maisha, Karma, Dominique, and I got wristbands, which felt so official, a signal that we belonged there. And we had a ball. We'd lie under beach umbrellas indulging in overpriced bar food served to us, interrupted only by refreshing dips in the pool and photoshoots with Kodak disposable cameras. We went to the casino in the resort, where I learned to play blackjack. No matter where we went or what we did that week, I found myself melting into the moment. *This must be what it feels like to relax*, I marveled at the realization. On the morning of our departure, we made a final trip into town, scouring the markets for the perfect thank-you gift for Maisha's aunt and uncle. Dominique, the consummate poet and writer, spotted a small glass figurine with four little birds perched on a branch, somewhat of an homage to Bob Marley's "Three Little Birds." We all signed the lovely letter she penned on our behalf and set out for our return to snowy Ann Arbor.

It was dark by the time we got back to campus, but I was

both relaxed and exhilarated. I floated into my dorm room; I couldn't wait to tell Leah all about the trip. Upon seeing that I had messages on my dorm phone, I slid out of my coat and dialed in to check them.

"Hey Daria, I know you're out of town, so call me when you get this. Something happened. I'm with Samuel." It was Leah. Her exhausted voice cut through the air.

Reality yanked me back to earth. What could have happened in the week I had been away? I called Samuel immediately, hoping to reach her. The moment he heard my voice, he handed her the phone.

"Hey, I got your message. What happened?"

"We got evicted. Mama is gone."

"WHAT? What do you mean?"

"I don't know. She's gone. I have no idea where she is. She's been gone for over a week at this point."

Questions flooded my mind, and I pointed the fire hose at her, spraying them all out. "Evicted? How? Wasn't she paying the rent? Where's Dr. Townsend? Wasn't he giving her money?"

The year we lived with Mr. Charles, my mother began to suffer chronic hip pain, a mysterious ailment for a thirty-seven-year-old. Eventually, she could barely walk without pain killers. We never went to the doctor, so when she made an appointment to see an orthopedic surgeon, I knew it was serious. Dr. George Townsend had determined that years of prednisone use, which she had been prescribed for sarcoidosis, ravaged her hip joints, resulting in avascular necrosis of the femur. Without cartilage, her hips had been reduced to "bone on bone," he said. She needed a bilateral total hip replacement.

Years later, I would research the link between sarcoidosis and drug use, if any, as well as the risk factors for developing avascular necrosis. In addition to steroid use, a common cause of avascular necrosis, heavy drinking is the leading cause, according to the Mayo Clinic. Smoking can also play a role. What I found most enlightening, though, is that years of cocaine and crack use can manifest in symptoms that mimic sarcoidosis.

During her several-months-long recovery from the surgery, my mother had gotten close to Dr. Townsend, and shortly into her rehabilitation, they began an affair, which lasted until after I left for college. I was furious that my mother would date a married man, especially one old enough to be her father. His wife managed his medical practice; we had seen this woman when we took my mother for pre- and post-op appointments. She answered his phones and filed patient medical records. She was the mother to his four adult children and, presumably, she raised them as he built his medical career. I was disgusted with him for being such a gross cliché.

Suddenly it all made sense. He had gotten us that apartment and had likely agreed to pay for it. They must have broken up, I concluded. It was the only explanation I could summon for how something like this could happen.

"They said the rent hasn't been paid for months," Leah reported. "I got a call at school from the management company the other day saying that I had a few hours to come get our stuff because they were going to throw it out on the street. By the time I got home, they had put everything out on the curb. I tried Dr. Townsend's office, but his wife answered the phone. I didn't speak to him. Then I called Dr. Ivery, and he sent movers to come get what was left and put it in storage. He said he'd pay for it to stay there for a few months while we figure out what to do."

I had been too disoriented by everything unfolding before me to be angry that she had called my boyfriend's father. I'm sure it was a last resort. I'm sure he expected my mother to show up and find the money to retrieve our things. I'm sure a part of me did too. Leah had managed to save some of our childhood photos and a few of her personal items. But I never saw my varsity jacket again, or my cheerleading and geometry trophies. My high school yearbooks, my prom dress—which Mrs. Ivery had gifted to me as a graduation present—were all gone. We had taken only what we could carry to Aunt Claudia's house. Now there was officially nothing left of my childhood. This may explain why I am hardly sentimental about things and have a disdain for hoarding. I'm a purger; most things just don't seem worth holding on to.

I had been away in an actual paradise while we were being evicted from our apartment. I was stunned. Who calls a high school student at school to tell them they're being thrown out? Was that supposed to have been considered a courtesy call? I don't remember how I actually responded. My sister would tell you that I muttered something to the effect of "This is insane. I'm just glad I wasn't there." We have fought many times over the years about this claim: her insistence that I was cold, callous, and self-interested in her time of greatest despair, and my refusal to believe that such a thought would have ever crossed my mind, let alone come out of my mouth. After all, I had been the one who—during my sophomore year of high school—worked as a waitress at the Bob's Big Boy in Fairlane Mall until 10 p.m. on school nights and then took the bus home late at night, and gave her bus fare for school most days because I had the fortune of carpooling to school with a classmate when we lived with Aunt Claudia. I all but did her algebra homework on more than one occasion when she grew disinterested. I made my father go with me to one of her track meets because I'd never had anyone come to my performances. I insisted that she go to college. I was the older sister. But that's what she believes she heard. I suppose it's possible that I blurted this out in the way one might say the most awkward thing at a funeral or when something so tragic happens and your brain is so frozen in shock that you fail to produce thoughts or words that make sense. It just doesn't sound like me to me.

Some say that grief is love with nowhere to go. But what happens when you must grieve a loss so many times that you become numb? My mother's recurrent disappearances had already inflicted an emotional whiplash. But this time was different. She had left us homeless, and it marked a fork in the road for how Leah's and my lives would unfold, the end of lives lived in parallel. Although my "home" was now confined to a single room in the Mary Markley Residence Hall, I lived on a beautiful campus where all of my needs were met, while Leah sought refuge with Samuel's mother, Linda, until she—unexpectedly pregnant—graduated from high school that summer. Within months, she and Samuel would get an apartment, get married, and have the baby shortly after Leah's eighteenth birthday. I had worked so hard to get out and was suddenly left with a desperate sense of helplessness, for not being able to take Leah with me when I left for college or to help her somehow when we lost the apartment— one that would haunt me for decades. Had Leah somehow become collateral damage to my need to leave?

Losing different mothers, we had different reactions. Leah always seemed to need her more than I did. At some point after my mother disappeared the second time, I confronted the possibility that perhaps she had died. Perhaps from an overdose, maybe foul play with the wrong crowd, or even suicide. My body had been present, but my spirit wandered, searching for the remnants of a family that had dissolved like salt in water. Yet, I refrained from delving too deeply into the realm of what-ifs. When more than a year had passed and she didn't even surface to meet her first granddaughter, it felt like a logical assumption. Still, there was no funeral, no official closure. Who would even make that call? With no proof of her fate, I was left with a most unique kind of grief: complex and disenfranchised. The isolation of my secrets was already so profound, and there was no literature or language to navigate the emotions tied to a mother who may or may not have died. In response, I chose to do what I believed she should have done when Grandma died—put my sadness in its "proper place," refusing to be consumed with the loss. *I* would not be defined by tragedy.

This perceived "death" brought an unexpected sense of freedom. Explaining why I didn't have a mother was tragic, but simple—she had died. I tested this narrative on classmates, finding solace in offering an answer that people could understand, even if it garnered the pity I loathed. She was better off gone, as far as I was concerned.

With my mother gone, I became further resolved in my plan to live differently. I doubled down on my life at school, burying this whole other part of me alive. I studied English literature and fantasized about becoming a novelist or a broadcast journalist. I would fall in love with musical theater after performing in *Godspell* and *Sweet Charity* while writing for the *Michigan Daily* arts section, meeting my work-study requirements, and working to graduate from college "with distinction" at twenty. In my pursuit of independence and a life divergent from the one I had growing up, my mother hunger fueled in me a relentless ambition.

My drive to excel went beyond survival; it was a Pavlovian coping mechanism—like dissociation—that kept me anesthetized to the feelings of abandonment and loss. But it also became a cage, keeping me disconnected from myself and from others.

There were moments where the armor gave way. During winter break of my sophomore year, I took a road trip with my friend Lauren. We became fast friends during my freshman year, bonding over our love of makeup, fashion, and music. We spent much of the ten-hour drive from Ann Arbor to Washington, DC, belting the lyrics to Whitney, Janet, and Mariah, and trading stories about all that we had going on as college students, from coursework to boy drama. As we approached Lauren's hometown of Reston, Virginia, we started talking about our early lives. *This is my chance*, I thought. *We're becoming good friends; I can tell her.*

I started slowly, sharing the surface-level parts of my story first. And then I dove into the darker details—how my parents were both addicts, the times I'd stolen food when we had none, how we'd often gone without heat or running water. I was nineteen and I'd never said any of this to anyone before. Lauren, who had lived a life of privilege, comfort, and access, fixed her eyes on me while I drove, my eyes remained fixed on the road. Seemingly in shock, she replied, "I thought you came from money!" I let out an awkward half laugh, unsure of how to respond. There was neither judgment nor pity in her voice. It wasn't that she saw me, but that she didn't see what I thought she would. And I felt relief. I appeared to belong in her world. I left Detroit as a girl who had only known scarcity and walked onto campus as someone with means. Not because I ever said it but because everyone believed it. My ability to blend in made me feel powerful, even if I had put my first crack in the veneer.

More than two years would pass before my mother resurfaced without a word—like a ghost—a week before my college graduation. In the time she had been away, Leah had two daughters and I had forged a path out of Michigan and toward my future. I was starting the next chapter of my new life, and I was too angry to let her anywhere near it. But as I built a life that distanced me from the circumstances and environment of my upbringing, the yearning for maternal guidance lingered beneath the surface. "Our maternal legacies, and the mitochondrial DNA that wires them into place, keep our mothers' voices alive within us in a particularly powerful way," explains Dr. Christine Northrup. Each achievement carried the weight of an unmet need for maternal affirmation. The wound of not being able to inspire my mother to treat me better was still there.

Another year and a half went by before I would slowly begin to construct a relationship with my mother for the first time as an adult, exclusively by phone. She had been back in Leah's life, performing an important familial role to her and her daughters. Newly single after a devastating breakup with my college boyfriend, I could no longer call on his family that had become like my own, and I felt alone. At twenty-two, I was living and working in Houston, where we'd moved after graduation, and my mother and I had not seen each other or spoken in nearly four years. I didn't know what we'd talk about, if we had anything in common, aside from our love of music and the dark circles that rest under the same stare. The unspoken disappearance lingered between us, and it seemed best to move forward without revisiting the past. Little did I know, the past was vividly present, and I had unknowingly been waiting for her to reclaim me.

She was marrying a man she had met the year before. She seemed stable; at the very least she had a home. We bonded over Leah's venture into motherhood, the mundane aspects of my work as a marketing coordinator at a local corporate and commercial architecture and interior design firm, and my consideration for whether I'd pursue a PhD in English literature having ruled out law school. It wasn't a nurturing relationship. There was no motherly advice, no guidance for how to think about my young adult life even in the simplest of ways. One thing had not changed: Even in her inability to help me steer in any particular direction, my mother always offered the same words when it came to pursuing my goals: "You can do anything you set your mind to." The reconnection was superficial, but hearing her voice provided me with a momentary relief that felt like whatever had been broken in me was slowly being knit back together. It wasn't much, but I had my mom back.

Despite a lack of evidence, I allowed myself to believe that she was finally sober and, with so many miles between us, that it was safe to introduce her to the twenty-two-year-old version of me. I wanted to believe that perhaps if she saw me, she'd be committed to change. I decided to go home to Detroit for Christmas that year, cautiously optimistic about seeing my mother for the first time in almost four years and meeting her new husband, Danny. I was staying at Leah's house for the holiday, so I drove to their house with my nieces, ages two and three, in tow. At sixteen months apart, the girls reminded everyone of me and Leah as kids.

I was relieved to see that they lived in a decent neighborhood and in a house far nicer than where I had grown up. It was a hopeful sign, a glimmer of the stability I had longed for her to find. The house, with its neat fence and the dog in the yard, symbolized a life that seemed normal. They had all been Danny's, but she had chosen to marry him, and that felt like something. I forgot about her surgery for a moment when she opened the door without her cane, until she limped as she walked toward us. It had only been a few years, but she seemed older. Or maybe more mature. She was clear-eyed, and there was something more settled about her, a semblance of peace I had not seen before.

I carried the baby on my left hip and held the toddler's hand with my right, the girls serving as an unintentional buffer, making a hug all but impossible. She helped me get them inside and as she greeted them, I could smell only her perfume. Issey Miyake. There wasn't the slightest hint of nicotine. I remembered that she'd quit smoking when she had the hip replacement.

The reunion went swiftly downhill, as my mother disappeared behind a locked door with Danny, promising they'd be "out in a minute." Thirty minutes passed, then an hour. I looked at the two little girls I'd brought into the situation, and I lost it. Shaking with rage, I screamed through the door, "We're leaving! I will never let you do to these girls what you did to me and Leah! And if I have my way, you'll never see them again." My words echoed in the silence that followed, a final, desperate plea for her to choose us.

When she finally emerged, I searched my mother's face for some sign of panic or regret that I was upset and abruptly ending the visit. Nothing. Instead, she said coolly, as if I were a little girl, "Daria, I told you we were coming right out. No need to be upset."

She had mastered the tone of a hostage negotiator, and I had forgotten how easily she could dismiss my feelings. She was the one in control, and I was the child who needed to regain her composure after a tantrum. The truth remained a stranger in the room, unwelcome in the company of denial. I felt woozy from the mindfuck she'd just pulled on me and nauseous from holding so much in. The only tears were mine. Everyone else stood in apparent confusion, almost as if they were embarrassed for me. But I was not confused. In fact, I had never seen more clearly. I was done, and this time, *I* was leaving *her.* That day in 2002 marks the last time I spoke to my mother. I was forced to abandon my fantasy of her sobriety, and I made the decision to walk away from the relationship that threatened to trap me, forever, in my childhood and in a state of extreme distress. I would never become the highest version of myself in the place that had threatened to destroy me.

8

DAMAGED PARTS

No one goes to a therapist for the first time when things are going great. It's more like a harrowing Saturday-morning "what have I done with my life" kind of decision. But that's exactly how my therapy journey began. At twenty-six, I was a second-year MBA student at the New York University Stern School of Business. As one of nine Black women in my class of over four hundred students, I had defied the odds to secure a coveted internship at L'Oréal, etching my name among the handful of Black women from NYU Stern to do so, and had received an offer to join their Luxury Products Division full-time after graduation. I had succeeded in doing the unthinkable. I was a world away from Detroit and on the path to success. I'd gotten out. I thought I was "done." I had made the painful but necessary decision to leave my mother behind and abandon all fantasies of having a relationship with her. I left the abused little girl in Detroit. I buried the abandoned and angry teenager somewhere on Michigan's campus. I cut off my damaged parts and left them in Texas without the painful acknowledgment of the self-imposed amputations that sought to escape the haunting memories. "The hard work is behind me," I thought. All I had to do now was get through my second year of grad school.

It never once occurred to me that I had healing to do. Not even when, in a fit of fright, I booked an appointment with a therapist at the NYU Student Health Center. As the new school year began, I found myself facing a familiar worry—the prospect of yet another graduation standing solitarily amid classmates and their celebrating families. So, nine months before my business school commencement, I decided I needed to talk to someone to avoid the trigger of another lonely ceremony.

My first impression of Meghan was that she looked a bit like Téa Leoni. More accurately, like she could be Téa Leoni's younger sister: tall, thin, and blonde, with a chin-length bob that framed crystal-blue eyes and an easy, natural beauty that said, "I didn't wake up like this, but I also didn't try very hard." A WASP-y kind of understated beauty you'd find in Wisconsin to capture in a J.Crew catalog. Meghan was in her early to mid-thirties and married (a newlywed, I assumed, as her paperwork and email address showed both maiden and married names, but never at the same time).

She explained that our session would be completely confidential and that she would be taking private notes solely for her own reference.

"Was there something in particular that brought you in to see me?"

"Well, I am starting my second year of business school, so I'll be graduating in May, and it dawned on me recently that this will be my second graduation where none of my family will be there, and I need a strategy for how to get in front of the inevitable questions from my classmates about why no one is there for me."

"Okay…" Meghan's pen hovered above the pad. "Are you comfortable sharing why no one will be there?"

I braced myself, instantly feeling a mix of anticipation and dread.

"I don't have parents. I mean, I do. They are alive. But they aren't in my life. I've been estranged from my mother for almost five years now and my father was always in and out of my life. More out than in. My parents split up when I was two, divorced when I was eight. They both have substance abuse problems. I didn't have proximity to my father's issues, but my earliest memory of my mother using cocaine is when I was about seven."

My mouth suddenly felt dry, and my throat tightened as I spoke, the words leaving a bitter aftertaste, vulnerability lingering on my tongue. The words hung in the room, a heavy confession that scratched the surface of a painful history, one I didn't have much practice speaking about.

Meghan's pen moved with grace. "What do you want to be able to say to your classmates?"

"Nothing, ideally. I used to wish I could just say that my parents were dead. Not because I wish they were, but because it would be so much easier. Of course, I could just say that I don't have a relationship with them or that they aren't in my life. But doesn't that seem weird? I don't know... not talking about them has generally been an effective strategy. Everyone talks about their family—what their parents do, where they're spending the holidays, their advice for how to think about recruiting. I just listen and never say anything about mine." It wasn't just the loneliness of graduations that brought me to her; it was the weight of this untold story.

"Is it possible that because you don't talk about your parents, people already have a sense that perhaps it's not something you want to talk about, so they don't ask?"

"Yeah, maybe."

With a gentle tone, Meghan offered, "So maybe there's nothing that you *have* to say about graduation either, unless you want to."

She wouldn't say it then, but Meghan determined that I had shown signs of C-PTSD, and she suggested that weekly cognitive behavioral therapy (CBT) sessions with her would be an approach to navigating the emotions being stirred by my impending graduation. Later, she would share her diagnosis, explaining that the emotions I sometimes wrestled with—those invisible anchors that seemed to pull me down at unexpected moments, the battles fought within the depths of my mind and body, where the echoes of trauma reverberate long after the wounds have healed—had a name: complex post-traumatic stress disorder.

"PTSD is the body continuing to defend against a threat that belongs in the past," explains Bessel van der Kolk in *The Body Keeps the Score*. And mine had the nerve to be complex.

While both PTSD and C-PTSD share roots in trauma, the latter emerges from a sustained exposure to the interpersonal horrors that leave indelible marks on the soul. Chronic childhood abuse, long-term captivity, or ongoing domestic violence birth C-PTSD, a condition made from trauma that is repetitive. As statistics offer a glimpse of the prevalence of PTSD—11 percent of people face the diagnosis in their lifetime, 3.5 percent of US adults annually—the gendered and racial contours of this affliction paint a grim tableau. Women are more susceptible than men, with Black, Latino, and Native Americans disproportionately burdened.

But the constellation of symptoms that persists months, sometimes years, beyond the inciting event with PTSD—intrusive thoughts, hyperarousal, flashbacks, nightmares and sleep disturbances, changes in memory and concentration and startle responses, distorted thoughts and feelings about oneself in relation to the cause of the event, or other behavior that can be described as easily irritable and reactive, paranoid, or reckless—is often more pervasive and enduring with C-PTSD, as the trauma is repetitive and complex. The only real description that resonated with me goes like this: "Having C-PTSD is like being homesick with no idea of what home is supposed to be." Longing for a place that doesn't exist.

Years later, I would come to understand that the impact of trauma resides in the limbic system, also known as the survival part of the brain. It detects threats and clings to a perpetual state of vigilance, amplifying fear responses to perceived traumas. It's like having eyes and ears everywhere. I can be engaged in a conversation with one person and hear everything the people next to me are discussing. I am guilty of toggling from my one conversation—mine—to another as if it were perfectly normal. Simultaneously, the limbic system stifles the prefrontal cortex, the command center for rationality and emotional regulation, in a silent betrayal of the very faculties that define humanity.

The day Meghan offered this observation, I sat there, absorbing the impact of her words. Complex post-traumatic stress disorder: branding me, tethering me to a past I had tried so desperately to escape—the raw, untamed wilderness of emotions that sprawled beyond clinical designations and diagnostic checkboxes. A shattered mirror, the sharp edges always threatening to cut, while reflecting a distorted image of the past. The term carried an unsettling sense of finality, as if it confirmed that I was forever marked by my experiences. It was a label that spoke of unspeakable horrors and invisible wounds, a name that held within it the history of a thousand battles and the promise of endless healing.

"What does that mean exactly?" I asked, my voice barely

above a whisper. Part of me feared her answer, afraid of what it might reveal about how much like my mother I actually was, about how delusional I had been to believe that leaving Detroit and walking away from her was all I had to do to be well, when they were only my first steps.

Meghan leaned forward slightly, her gaze steady and compassionate. "It means that the trauma you experienced during your childhood has left a lasting impression on your mental and emotional well-being."

By then I was sobbing and could hardly grasp my breath. My heart throbbed, a migraine in my chest. "I...I can see that...Will I always have it? Can it be cured?"

"You may feel like you are in a state of healing for a long time, but of course it can be treated. Our time together, even this moment right now, we are managing it."

"I spent all of these years trying to not be defined by my past and you're telling me that it's actually running my life? And that I have to relive it to get past it? What if I'm not strong enough?"

My childhood, as I saw it, was a burden that bore all of the pain I had been given that was never mine to carry. I resisted the feelings of loss, mourning, and shame, and my response was to further dissociate. I bisected my identity: There was the Daria who had grown up in Detroit and the Daria who had gotten out. The first part of me had no connection to the second. I saw my past as if it had happened to someone else. I learned to leave my body the night my mother's boyfriend Tim called for me to sit on his lap while he watched TV in the dark living room and, after I nodded off to sleep, touched me over my pajama bottoms. I awoke to his left hand between my legs and his right hand on himself, over his jeans. I froze, pretending to stay asleep while creating a plan for how I'd get away. I decided that I would "wake up" with a very big gesture and insist that it was my bedtime, allowing me to run upstairs and go to bed. I avoided Tim for the months that he and my mother remained together, a sufficient enough tactic to evade another encounter. I never told my mother about it. It didn't seem worth mentioning. Dissociation wasn't the result of a scary science experiment or a freaky out-of-body experience; it was a cashmere blanket and a glass of wine in front of a cozy fire.

By twenty-six, I had a fully formed thesis that my most protected self was the one that had been separated from this incessant assault on my sense of security.

Together, Meghan and I explored the ways in which C-PTSD had insidiously shaped my responses to the world—the hypervigilance born from a childhood of unpredictable danger, the fear of attachment rooted in the repeated betrayals of my mother—all had been embedded in me. In new surroundings, I found myself searching for potential threats that weren't there. I craved connection, but the fear of being let down, abandoned, or worse lingered like a silent warning, so I often chose to withdraw.

But what I feared most was not an external threat

waiting to pounce from the periphery. The real fear gnawed at the edges of my consciousness, urging me to keep moving, keep pushing—against the constraints of time, ambition, and even geography. Higher, faster, further—I became a relentless traveler in perpetual motion, as if standing still would awaken the very thing I had eluded. That it would devour me the moment I stopped. Meghan would help me see that I could never outrun it. That the thing I was most afraid of being caught by was already there. *That's what you get for thinking you're special. You aren't special. You ain't shit.* That voice, echoing in my head, quick and severe. Brutal.

No longer consumed with the demands of basic survival, I could suddenly hear it everywhere—the one that interrupted my thoughts, the one that commented every time I saw myself in the mirror or criticized me when I made a mistake. The litany of lies unfurled.

You should have been better. If you were, your mother would have chosen to be there for you. You weren't worth the hard work of getting sober. She didn't really want you. She told you that lie when she was feeling generous and wanted to show you kindness. When she said she wished she'd aborted you, that was the truth. You were a burden. If your own parents didn't want you, what makes you think anyone else does?

Trauma, that masterful storyteller, had woven a web of lies, and armed with evidence gathered over the years, I had become a reluctant believer. These untruths, insidious and cunning, had rooted themselves deep in me, distorting perceptions and recycling a narrative that said that my worthiness hinged on the power to change the unchangeable. If only I were enough, the story insinuated, the world around me would shift, my mother would change, the wounds of the past would miraculously heal. The lie seduced me into a futile dance of self-blame and self-improvement, obscuring the truth that my intrinsic value transcended external circumstances. Trauma, the artful architect of such stories, told me tales of abandonment, unworthiness, and irreparable brokenness. Tales that had unknowingly become the foundation of my identity and had imprisoned me in a warped reality.

As Meghan helped illuminate the darkest corners of my mind, she assured me that I was not subject to a life sentence in some biological prison, that the past need not dictate my future, that reliving it wouldn't break me, that I could survive my feelings and live with the truth, whatever it was. "Only if you let it," she affirmed, recognizing the resilient core within me. "And knowing you, you aren't going to let that happen."

I nodded through my tears. It made sense. I wasn't yet convinced, but it made sense.

Our sessions that first year laid bare the impact of my life so far being predicated on abuse and neglect. Meghan helped me not to shy away from the darkness that I worked to bury; instead she encouraged me to lean into it, to explore its depths with curiosity and compassion. Healing would begin with acknowledgment, an honest confrontation with the wounds I carried, a recognition of the pain that lingered beneath the surface. I began lifting the layers of gauze that covered them, staring at the gaping holes wondering where to start. I tore open every emotional wound, all of which I'd spent the preceding two decades numbing. I was forced to revisit places in my memory and the disowned parts of myself that threatened to break me open. But it was a hole I had to climb through.

As graduation approached, my anxiety shifted from how I would manage that day to how I would manage without Meghan. I would no longer be a student and, therefore, unable to continue on under her care. Before I could ask her for recommendations for other therapists in New York City, she announced that she had news.

"I have decided to leave NYU and go into private practice at the end of the school year."

"Wait, that means I can keep seeing you after I graduate!"

"Yes, if you'd like to continue working together, we will be able to do so."

I would embark on a journey with Meghan, a pilgrimage through the layers of dissociation, acknowledgment, and integration, every week for nearly five years, the start of my almost two decades of therapy. That painful but necessary step of excavating the experiences of my childhood and early adult life remains the most meaningful step in meeting my own interiority.

9

PERFECTLY REAL

One night during my first year of business school, I turned to Jake while in bed at my East Village studio apartment and asked, "Do your parents know about me?" I wasn't just asking if they knew he was seeing someone; I wanted to know if they knew I was Black. We'd been together for four months, and it seemed like a fair question.

"Of course they know about you." He coughed up a laugh. And then proceeded to tell me about the two-page email of meticulously outlined disapproval in which his mother invited him to contemplate how difficult it would be for an interracial couple in the world, urged him to consider the many challenges mixed-race children face, and pleaded with him to be careful if we were "intimate" because I'd likely try to get pregnant.

My heart pounded with defiance. "She *does* know that I'm your classmate at Stern, right? And that I'm interning at

L'Oréal this summer? And that I got better grades than you did in college? And graduated in three years? And that I got into Columbia Business School when you didn't? Who do your parents think you're dating?!"

"Hey"—he reached for my hand, his thumb brushing mine—"it's upsetting to me, too. I'm really caught off guard here. I obviously don't agree with them. They're just showing concern the way they know how. My mom said a lot of the mixed-race kids in her class struggle the most and she'd hate to see us go through that."

"Struggle how? Go through what?"

"I don't know, Daria. They just have their concerns."

I felt a surge of determination. *Challenge accepted*, I thought, convinced my accomplishments would mean something in a world where the color of my skin still spoke louder than anything I could ever say. "Well, they haven't met me yet," I said, my voice steady despite the storm brewing inside.

But there was another layer—the familiar dread that came with revealing my family situation. Jake was only the third man I'd had to explain it to, and every time, I worried about the right moment to break the news. Worried that when they learned I wasn't the "girl next door" I appeared to be, they'd decide that I wasn't worth the trouble.

The invitation to spend Thanksgiving in Pennsylvania with Jake's family came with unsettling anxiety. Meeting the parents for the first time is a big step in any relationship. I had always done so successfully—parents loved me—but this time felt even more significant. Jake assured me that his family was open-minded and looking forward to meeting me, but I couldn't shake the unease I felt as we made our way to the house. As we pulled up to the picturesque Tudor tucked into their cul-de-sac, I took a deep breath and plastered a smile on my face. Together we stepped out of the car; I cradled a bouquet of flowers I'd bought, hopefully, for the center of the table. Jake carried the bottles of wine. He squeezed my hand reassuringly as we approached the front door.

Thanksgiving at the Bowen house was a master class in restrained civility. As we entered their home, Jake's parents greeted us with smiles that failed to reach their eyes—a veneer of welcome over foundations of doubt. I studied the mélange of aromas, the sage-laden stuffing and the warmth of pumpkin pie, hoping they might soften the edges of this encounter.

Then came dinner, the moment I had been both anticipating and dreading. Jake's younger brothers were there along with their long-term girlfriends, the promise of a built-in buffer. Still, as we gathered around the table, engaging in conversation, I couldn't shake the feeling of being under scrutiny. Jake's mother, in particular, seemed to watch me with a keen eye.

"Does anyone like dark meat?" Jake's dad asked as he stood carving the turkey.

"I don't mind it," Jake chimed in. I looked at him and a laugh escaped me.

As we passed the dishes around the table, everyone started to share their Thanksgiving favorites.

Shit. Mine aren't here. What am I going to say?

When it was my turn, I said something to the effect of, "It would be hard to choose between collard greens and macaroni and cheese…but…mashed potatoes and gravy are definitely a close third."

"Oh! I don't think I've ever had collard greens before," his father said in a slightly northern West Virginia accent, the twang likely softened by decades in DC. "But it's probably a lot like spinach, I'd guess?"

"Hmm." I paused, actually thinking about it. "I guess if you cooked spinach all the way down, the texture would be similar. Not sure I can really liken greens to anything else, though. Maybe kale? They have an earthier flavor. And the preparation is quite different." I couldn't help but feel displaced and separate from everyone else at the table.

Over the course of the evening, I pirouetted through topics from my time at Michigan to business school, to having also lived in DC before moving to NYC to attend NYU, to my internship at L'Oréal and my plans to go back after graduation. Each contribution garnered the subtlest of responses that chafed against my skin. My words were met with nods, the kind that acknowledge rather than approve. I could feel the invisible checklist they held between us, each of my achievements weighed and found wanting.

They didn't even serve macaroni and cheese to soften the landing.

Three days with Jake's family was exhausting. I felt like

I'd been auditioning for seventy-two hours straight. The day after we'd gotten back to New York, I asked him what his parents thought of me, to which he only replied, "My mother said you were a great conversationalist."

I smiled and said something along the lines of "That's nice of her to say," but inside, I felt deeply disappointed. Had there been more, he would have been excited to tell me. She had basically given a less microaggressive equivalent of "She's so articulate."

After Thanksgiving with Jake's family, I looked for a glimmer of hope—a sign, however small, that perhaps, with time and understanding, we might find a way to bridge the gap between his family and me and build a deeper connection based on acceptance and, eventually, love. There were times it felt possible, like when his parents came to NYC to visit and saw the apartment we shared in Chelsea or the Christmas when they'd hung a stocking for me next to Jake's. But mostly, I found myself faltering under the pressure of their expectations to magically one day show up as someone I would never be. It took me a long time to see that it was not just their approval I sought; it was affirmation that I mattered. That my efforts to make myself into someone lovable weren't in vain. Staying in that relationship for as long as I did now feels like an act of self-betrayal at best and self-hatred at worst.

But I had bought into the myth of Black exceptionalism, that I had checked off the boxes that made me somehow "the right kind of Black girl": "twice as good" (as the average white person); and the best at any table worth joining. The unintended implication is that we aren't enough as we are.

When my oldest niece, Aurora, turned thirteen, I flew her out to New York from Detroit for a weekend celebration. I wanted to honor this "big age" and celebrate her with a weekend that was just about her. I had everything planned. Rory would get to the city Thursday evening, and I would order dinner to be delivered to my apartment while we caught up. Friday morning, I'd let her sleep in, something that she rarely got to do as the oldest of four. We'd have a slow morning followed by an early lunch before some shopping, and that evening, we'd have a proper dinner out. On Saturday, we had tickets to the matinee performance of *Wicked* on Broadway—based on one of our favorite books. Afterward, we'd do a little more shopping on Fifth Avenue, eventually reaching our destination, Tiffany & Co., where I would get her a sterling silver necklace with an initial charm to commemorate the trip and her milestone birthday.

Hours before her arrival, I got an email that was going to blow up the start of the weekend. I had been going back and forth with a woman at *O, The Oprah Magazine* about a potential partnership, and she finally confirmed a time to meet— Friday at 11 a.m. I confirmed and explained that I would have my niece with me and asked if it would be okay for her to wait for me in the lobby during the meeting.

"Of course—that's totally fine," she replied. "Just send

me her name and I'll make sure you're both registered with security."

I fussed over what Rory wore, wanting to make sure she was "appropriately" dressed. Of course she hadn't packed anything "dressy." She was thirteen. *I* was the adult with the meeting. Why did it matter what she wore? But I fussed. I wish I hadn't now. I would have never wanted to make her feel like what she brought wasn't good enough. Like *she* wasn't good enough. The thought alone brings me to tears. We went through everything she had packed and decided on a top that worked under a black cardigan I owned. I also gave her a pair of Kate Spade earrings and my black puffer to wear. New York wasn't colder than Detroit, but she hadn't packed for walking around outside in January.

We arrived at Hearst Tower, checked in, and headed up to the O floor. We were greeted by the woman I was meeting, and as she heard me telling my niece to wait in the lobby and that I'd be back shortly, she chimed in.

"Would you like to see the fashion closet?" she asked.

Rory looked at me for the okay. I smiled and said, "How cool is that? Do you want to see it?"

"Oh my God! Yes, please!" she said.

"Great! You just can't take or post pictures of anything, okay?" the woman cautioned.

"Yes, of course!"

Back at my apartment later that afternoon, my niece said, "Auntie, you're Superwoman."

High praise from her has always meant the world to me. Even today, nothing makes me prouder than when Rory thinks I've done something cool. I value her judgment and respect her mind. She's one of my favorite people in the world.

"I am not," I assured her humbly, although my ego loved the idea that she saw me that way. I didn't even know exactly what I had done to earn the title, but I didn't want to play into the idea that Black women are superheroes or that she had to do any of the things I'd done to be seen as strong.

"Well, I think you are," she insisted.

"Thanks, doll. The trick is," I began, "to find the things you do really well and do them as much as you can. There are plenty of things I don't do well. I just don't spend much time or energy on them." Today, I can't help but think of it as my ego's way of saying "I play small to avoid feeling small." I didn't know then that what I was afraid of had no business running my life.

I remember at the time feeling very satisfied with my response, as though I had imparted some great wisdom to Rory. My intended message was "Play to your strengths." This I still believe. (Studies have shown that we are much more fulfilled at work and in life when we do strengths-based work.) But a subtext also existed, an underlying message that suggested "Do only the things that make you look good to other people, and you will be deemed wonderful."

Perfectionism comes in the fear of not being good enough

disguised as the pursuit of being the best. It promises that it's virtuous, that it's the quest for excellence. And in it, I got lost. It was a sneaky kind of self-sabotage, an unsustainable balancing act between ambition and exhaustion as I pushed myself to excel beyond measure. It was the high bar I set—a standard so pristine, so impossibly polished, that it glinted in the sun like a blade, and I skated its edge, terrified to slip. I constantly looked to others for cues that I was "doing it right." I told myself that if I could just get it right, I would be safe from criticism, from rejection, from the very essence of being human, which is to be beautifully flawed. And in so doing, all I did was paint myself into a corner, a porcelain doll on the shelf, afraid to move, to breathe, to truly live.

Given my career choice, people often ask about my passion for beauty—when it was born and how I made the decision to nurture it. As a girl, I saw beauty as elusive, something that only a handful of the world's most fortunate were born with. And according to my mother, I was not one of those lucky few. My self-consciousness about my looks started when I was about five, initiated by my mother's incessant criticisms about my nose, which was too short and wide, with prominent nostrils. My mother would take a wooden clothespin—the ones Grandma used to hang laundry outside on hot summer days—and clip it over my button nose. She hoped that the constant pinching would cinch just the right spot, making it narrower, like hers. For my mother, "famous" for her beauty in her own little world, pretty was important. Having an average-looking daughter simply wouldn't do.

She later turned to my hair, which didn't have the same smooth, wavy texture or length as my sister's or that of my grade school classmate Lana Colston, who had a Black mother and an East Indian father. Later still, it was my breasts, which developed quickly and began to sag before I left high school. "Anything over a mouthful is a waste," she would say in her own defense when the question was raised of how I wound up with big boobs when my mother and sister had not. Most girls cringed at the thought of going to shop for training bras with their mothers. Instead, I begged mine for one until she took me to Target and bought the first bra that appeared to be my size.

I used to wonder if "pretty" was contagious. If, by osmosis, I could be as beautiful as my mother or Lana or the girls I'd study in the magazines I read. I wondered if using Lana's hairbrush would magically transform my fuzzy ponytail into long silky strands that would cascade down my back. I chastised my reflection, praying to God that I would wake up a stunning beauty, or at least, one of those people who "grew into their looks." Any beauty I had, I concluded, would be an act of self-creation. And I had more than enough ambition and discipline to make it happen.

Having learned to see myself through my mother's eyes, I devoted countless hours to the artistry of my appearance— meticulously arranging my hair and makeup before venturing out for the simplest of errands. I would earn every compliment I received. If I felt less than, plagued by a sense of inadequacy over my appearance or my wardrobe, I chose isolation over the possibility of joy, even if it meant missing an event I was excited to attend. I once canceled my own birthday celebration ninety minutes before I was scheduled to meet up with twenty friends after the place I'd carefully chosen closed unexpectedly and I couldn't find a suitable alternative. I stayed home and lamented over the failure of the night, unwilling to settle for "some shitty bar" in the Village. I was a statue in my own life, often observing but not participating, feeling the world move around me in a blur of colors and sounds to which I had little claim.

"Don't fuck up, DB" had become a mantra.

"I don't feel like a three-dimensional person," I said to Meghan one session. I had been in a state of constant chase, lost in standards I didn't create for myself. In hindsight, I was running more than chasing. Still, the one-dimensional pursuit of excellence was taking a psychological toll.

"When you think about yourself separate from the things you've achieved and the roles you fill," she began, her voice a gentle nudge toward introspection, "who are you without those things? Who are you without your résumé?"

"I'm not sure," I admitted. "Growing up, I was 'the smart one.' I didn't have much of a perception of myself outside of achieving, of doing well in school. I was good at being good. But there weren't other attributes or aspects of my personality that were highlighted as positive that I was encouraged to nurture. I was a ham, quite a goofy kid, if you can believe it. And my mother used to always say, 'I hope you grow out of this silly stage.' That's all I remember."

"I want you to ask someone close to you how they see you, separate from what you've achieved. It can be enlightening to see ourselves through the eyes of those who know us beyond our accomplishments."

The task felt a little daunting, but it seemed like a great idea. Later that evening, I decided to ask Jake.

"If you took my résumé and all of my accomplishments away, who am I?"

"That's a silly question," he laughed. "Why would I separate you from what you've achieved? They make you who you are."

His words, meant to reassure, instead echoed my fear.

"No, seriously. I talked about this in therapy with Meghan today, and she suggested that I ask you. So, who am I, without all that?" I pressed, needing him to understand.

"It's really hard to isolate certain aspects of a person that are part of who they are. You are driven and ambitious. Those are good things. You've overcome a lot to get where you are, which makes you determined. But I'd also say, you can have a conversation with almost anyone, and you have a good eye for things—clothes, decorating...I don't know... Does that answer your question?"

The only thing it told me was that I had unwittingly

chosen someone who was happy to let me hide. Either he didn't think there was much more to me, or he couldn't be bothered to coax more out of me. I had allowed him to be a witness to my entire life, and myself to be steeped in his, and this was it?

Meanwhile, I had become the emblem for all the ways Jake had changed. Never mind the fact that he was the one who had uprooted his life for the cutthroat world of New York investment banking, carefully crafting his image to fit the mold; the tailored suits, the right haircut, the curated circle of acquaintances—all hallmarks of his ambition. I think I was the only person from Stern that he hung out with who was not in high finance. But sure, his preference for wine over beer and Aruba over Dewey Beach were a referendum on my influence. I soon became the Bowen family's scapegoat for his departure from the familiar. I'd somehow gotten caught in the middle of the negotiation between the person he was becoming and the one they wanted him to be.

The strain escalated and Jake handled it poorly. His method of coping was silence—a barrier that grew sturdier with each anxious attempt I made to close the widening gap between us.

My resentment grew stronger. I was staying to prove that I wasn't a runner. That I could commit to dealing with hard things and seeing this through to better times.

"He's emotionally constipated," I once told Meghan. "Ingrown, like a toenail." I thought of James Baldwin. "That family is so repressed. They don't ever talk about anything real. Nothing breaches the surface—weather, sports, the mundane cycle of current events." My therapy sessions increasingly centered on Jake's aversion to communication and depth, the strain of his family dynamics, my choice of an emotionally unavailable partner, and the looming question of whether I should remain in the relationship.

On the night I resolved to leave, I had been trying to get Jake to talk about something, and true to form, he shut down. By then, we were also seeing a couple's therapist, something I'd begged him to do for close to a year. He still had not found one for himself. We'd gotten into bed and, exhausted, I turned my back to him, resigned to get some sleep. Through tears I heard myself say the thing that shook me wide-awake:

"Trying to get you to talk to me...I feel like I did when I was a little girl and I used to write these letters to my mom... telling her that I knew she was sick, asking her to let me help her...Part of me thought she might get angry, storm out of her room, and curse me out or beat me, but she never did. She never said anything. Like it never happened. I feel like I'm back there with her."

My words had become a message across decades, unheard then, unheard now. It wasn't just Jake's silence that echoed my mother's; it was my own.

Two weeks later, I moved out.

10

FILTERED

S tay ahead of the pain. You don't want to be chasing it,"
my dentist once warned me after extracting all four
wisdom teeth, two of which were deeply impacted. I would
receive the same advice from my orthopedic surgeon after
he repaired two broken fingers a decade later.

I received no such warning with therapy. No heads-up
about the peculiar precision to the pain, a sharpness that
cuts more accurately than any scalpel. This precision is not
wielded with malevolence, but with the hope of excision, of
cutting away the diseased parts to allow for healing. Yet the
act of cutting, no matter how well intentioned, is an act of
violence against the self, a necessary brutality. But in this dil-
igent excavation, there is no anesthetic. The pain feels fresh,
as if the events of my childhood happened mere moments
ago. Memories once dulled by the passing of time sharpen
again, their edges cutting into the flesh of now, bleeding

into the everyday. The bleeding is not without purpose. It is the bloodletting of the mind, a release of the poison that has accumulated over years of untreated injuries. Still, the process is fraught with danger. The risk of infection is high.

I approached therapy with the same fervor that characterized my all-or-nothing approach to life. Barring vacations and her maternity leave, I faithfully showed up for weekly sessions with Meghan, availing myself completely to the task of "doing the work." I had gone beneath the surface and into the crevices where pain lived dormant, but very much alive. As the wounds were exposed, so too were my feelings: unprocessed and overwhelming.

In this quiet search for healing, we expose our most tender wounds to another's gaze and to our own, hoping that the fresh air will somehow carry away the pain. There is a particular kind of bravery required to lay your inner life open in this way, to let someone see you unguarded, with all the parts you'd rather hide laid bare. This exposure is a double-edged sword; it promises liberation and threatens devastation. The therapist's room, an asylum of sorts, is also a stage upon which we perform our deepest fears and sorrows, hoping the act of naming them will strip them of their power. There, the armor required for my high-octane life could be shed, layer by fragile layer. My wounds and I could breathe. But as soon as I went back into the world, back into my "real" life, the mask went back on.

That mask had become a surrogate, a persona onto

whom I could project the best versions of the various selves that existed—sister, friend, marketing executive, survivor. It clung to me like a heavy second skin, as if I was fighting against an invisible force that wanted to suffocate me. It obscured my vision, leaving me to stumble through those years, blinded by the smokescreen I had constructed. Putting blinders on had served me well, even if it meant shutting a part of the world out and a part of myself off. I saw it as a necessary deception in a life that was both public and private, where success hinged on the ability to seem unbroken, and every day was a performance for an audience too distracted to look closer.

My solution had been to embrace a work hard, play hard kind of life that kept me from going too deep for too long. In the city that never sleeps, I was perpetually awake, caught in a whirlwind of exclusivity and prestige—from employee-only invites to designer sample sales and New York Fashion Week events, to speaking on panels at top business schools across the country about what was considered a nontraditional post-MBA career path. I was so often onstage at Harvard, Columbia, Brown, and NYU that I earned the nickname "Keynote" from a group of Stern students in the graduating class three years after mine. These were the distractions that made the mask easier to bear.

On the surface, my life seemed enviable—vacations in Napa, Miami, Paris, and no shortage of social obligations that kept me too busy to face my pain. Each event was an invitation to compartmentalize the work I had done in therapy, while avoiding the truth of fear masquerading as ambition, of numb feelings parading as success.

Two months after breaking up with Jake and moving back to the Upper West Side, the winds of change had swept me up yet again, this time ushering me through the revolving doors of 767 Fifth Avenue—facing three of New York City's most esteemed landmarks: Bergdorf Goodman, the Plaza hotel, and Central Park. At thirty years old, I left Rent the Runway, where I had been the company's tenth employee, and became a director at the Estée Lauder Companies, leading marketing for the namesake brand's $350 million North American makeup business. "Director" wasn't just a title; it was a mantle I wore with a pride both genuine and performed.

As the world's fourth-largest prestige beauty brand, Estée Lauder had significant advertising budgets. And as a director of one of said budgets, the invitations flowed like champagne: lunches at Barney's (RIP), cocktail parties at Hearst Tower and on the Hudson River. Twice a year, we flew to Palm Beach and Scottsdale for our spring and fall sales conferences, where I'd stand onstage in front of several hundred Estée Lauder corporate and field executives to present product launch and marketing plans for the upcoming season. In Palm Beach, we celebrated a great first day of presentations on the lawns of the Lauder family estates.

To be in the realm of the Lauder family is to find oneself in the spectacle of a kind of American royalty. The Estée

Lauder offices are a world unto itself, a microcosm of legacy and opulence, where the weight of a family name carries with it the heft of history and Picasso and Braque adorned the office walls. It was one thing to meet with Aerin Lauder in her fortieth-floor office to discuss a product launch, but another altogether to tour the intimate spaces of their homes, where business mingled with personal, and a little brown glass bottle of Advanced Night Repair sat atop her dresser. To be ushered into the inner sanctum of the Lauder dynasty felt like stepping onto a stage set by generations of unassailable prestige.

The first time I attended the Breast Cancer Research Foundation's Hot Pink Party, I was breathless. It was a fundraiser for the world's largest private funder of breast cancer research, yes, but also a pageant of sorts, a celebration of fame and power dressed in philanthropy's garb. My title had earned me an invitation to this world, my role in the theater of the beautiful and the powerful. I remember glancing over at Zac Posen, who sat at the table next to mine, while a week at Donna Karan's Turks and Caicos home was being auctioned off. Sting took the stage, followed by a performance from Sir Elton John, and I went home in awe.

But the brightness was also blinding, and in the solitude of my own reflection, the heaviness always returned. The shadows of a self not fully realized waited patiently for the parties to end, for the mask to crack. In quiet moments, when the glitter settled and I slowed to stillness, the mask would slip, revealing a woman caught between the world she lived in and the truths she was trying to live with.

The external world demands continuity after all. It requires us to fulfill our roles and obligations, to function within the parameters set by society. Our culture fails to recognize our pain as an invitation to grow. Instead, it rushes to soothe and suppress, urging us back to a semblance of normalcy. "Normal" is the goal, but that's just code for anything that's considered socially acceptable, not spiritually enriched, not psychologically whole, not even personally fulfilled. Success became my shield, a way to deflect from the void within, one that therapy had begun to expose. This wasn't dissociation. It was more like avoidance laced with denial.

But in therapy, I was learning how to live alongside the pieces of myself I had tried so hard to forget. That pain didn't need to be a villain. It could be a compass, pointing to a part of me that could be acknowledged and contained, a quiet presence that I could choose to carry without letting it define me.

I pressed my palm against the cool wood, steeling myself for the plunge into familiar waters. The click of the door to Meghan's office, as it shut behind me, seemed less an echo and more a sealing off from the pulse of New York City I'd left on the concrete below. The room, with its deliberate calm, soft lighting casting a gentle glow over the walls, and thoughtfully chosen pillows and plants, offered comfort. The clock ticked, a reminder that time here moved differently, measured not in minutes but in revelations and reckonings.

"I have some news," Meghan said toward the end of the session, her voice carrying the same calm it always did, yet beneath it, something else—a reluctance perhaps. I sensed the nature of her news; I already knew she was pregnant with her second child. I braced myself for what was to come.

"This is really hard. I have not been looking forward to this conversation, but I will be leaving New York." The words, simple in their construction, carried the heaviness of an ending.

I tried to summon a response, something gracious or at least coherent, but the words dissolved before they could reach my lips.

"My husband got an exciting job opportunity," she continued, her voice laced with a tinge of excitement shadowed by the bittersweet undertone of departure. "And we are moving to Los Angeles." The complexity of her emotions mirrored my own—a mixture of joy for her and a selfish despair for my loss.

"Wow, that's...big news," I managed, the words feeling hollow, inadequate. "Huge. When are you leaving? Will you practice there? I have so many questions."

"We're leaving next month, so we have a few more weeks. I'll eventually practice there, but I'm going to take some time." She smiled, touching her belly with maternal affection. "We'll need to settle in and then this little guy will be here in a few months."

"Yes, of course, that makes sense. It's a big move and a busy time!"

"I know this might feel overwhelming," she continued, her empathy a light salve; it could scarcely heal the sudden rift her departure would create. "And I want you to know how incredibly proud I am of the work you've done."

"Thank you," I said, the gratitude heavy in my throat. "I'm going to miss you," I admitted, the confession feeling like a crossing of boundaries, a betrayal of some unspoken rule.

"I'm going to miss you too."

"Would it be okay to give you a hug?" I asked, recognizing the breach this would create in our relationship as therapist and patient.

"Of course," she said, and stood with an openness that invited the crossing of that line. It was a gesture of human connection that, for a moment, transcended the role she played in my life.

I would ordinarily have taken the subway home, but it was June, and the city already started to brew with enough humidity that made the idea of a thirty-minute subway ride unappealing. I knew a walk would do me some good, a chance to chew on and attempt to digest the news that Meghan was leaving. I left Union Square, heading north up Fifth Avenue, with a vague plan to take 21st Street west toward Sixth Avenue. My route wasn't deliberate; it was the path I always took, muscle memory guiding me to the apartment I once shared with Jake. A wave of nausea buckled my knees mid-stride, a visceral reaction to the upheaval of Meghan's news. In a moment of self-preservation, I hailed a taxi home to 77th Street, avoiding the anxiety of potentially running into him on the street, a reminder of another loss.

The taxi ride was a blur, the city passing by in a smear of lights and shadows. I tipped the driver more out of habit than gratitude and stepped out into the evening air, which had started to cool but still held the day's breath. The doorman greeted me with his usual chatty cheerfulness, but his words were lost to me, mere background noise to the uproar in my mind.

My apartment now felt less like a sanctuary and more like an oversized mausoleum for all the versions of myself I thought I had buried, and I was a ghost wandering through its former life. The living room blurred as tears welled up and spilled onto my cheeks, into my lap, down my blouse. Meghan had been the lighthouse guiding me through the treacherous waters of my past, and now she was leaving. *Meghan was leaving me.* The thought left me without an anchor in a sea of uncertainty. "How can I do this without you?" I cried into the void, a pitiful sound voicing the fear that gnawed at me. It wasn't just about her departure; it was about confronting the many aspects of healing I had yet to grasp. Meghan had ushered me through emotional upsets and awakenings, especially the end of my four-year relationship with Jake. And now, mere months after my breakup, she was leaving. I hadn't learned not to hold on so tight. I had only learned how to let go.

In some ways, I emerged from the process feeling more wounded, overwhelmed by the psychic toxins that therapy had released into my bloodstream. I was wholly unprepared for all that would come up and unsure of how I was supposed to manage it all on my own. Even with Meghan's referrals, the thought of starting over, of auditioning strangers to hold my most fragile truths, felt overwhelming. Regulating my nervous system—this flood of cortisol and fear—I hadn't yet learned how to do.

My expertise in detachment had given me a distance, a means to observe my life with a dispassionate curiosity, as one might a character in a novel. It had become both a shield and a telescope—offering protection and perspective yet keeping me at a distance from the raw intensity of my emotions. Get too close and you lack perspective. There is no margin when the image is full bleed on the page. This narrative farsightedness allowed the cool appraisal from afar. From there, I could see the contours of my sadness without being swallowed by it.

But therapy had required a haunting recitation that began with a trembling voice and grew firmer with each fifty-minute session. I was no longer insulated from the profound sense of abandonment, the kind of soul-crushing loneliness that compelled me to push the world away, even as I feared being discarded. An unwanted possession. Good for nothing. I was most often confronted by the things my mother made me believe about myself, including that my worth was measured by my usefulness to her and my ability to dazzle others. My needs did not matter. "Can anyone love me when my own mother doesn't? Would anyone choose to stay if my own parents hadn't?" ricocheted within me, questions that bled into the universe and returned with a chilling silence that sounded much like "no." It was like standing in quicksand; the more I struggled against this belief, the deeper I sank into it. I had unearthed every last hurt, dragging them out into the open, where they cluttered around me, a disorganized array of pain and confusion. And there I was, at the center of it all, paralyzed by the chaos of my own history, unsure of where to begin the process of reassembly.

For months after Meghan left, I would often wake to the familiar sensation of a knot in my stomach. I'd lie in bed trying to comb through the snarls of my discomfort, the physical from the emotional, but they were knotted too tightly together. Getting out of bed felt like a concession to the day more than a victory over the night. I moved through my morning rituals with mechanical obligation, performed with a detachment that was both deliberate and protective. My commute became a daily struggle. My tardiness at work eventually caught the attention of my VP, another reminder of the facade I was struggling to maintain. I brushed off his concerns with a promise that it wouldn't happen again, retreating further into my shell of avoidance.

It felt like a prolonged illness, one for which the cure was as distressing as the disease itself. A private agony, an unremitting, soul-deep migraine that threatened to extinguish the very essence of who I was. An invisible affliction, the kind in which the world becomes too glaring and too loud and you're left clutching your head in a desperate bid for silence, for any kind of reprieve. Surviving it didn't feel like strength; it felt like luck. The fact that my depression didn't kill me, a mystifying miracle, left me standing, however unsteadily, bewildered by my own survival.

11

WISDOM OF THE WOUND

The early Saturday morning light spilled over my notes, casting long shadows across the words that were supposed to bridge the gap between who I was as a girl and who I had become. My hands shuffled through the note cards, aligning the edges with a precision I demanded from everything. I glanced at my reflection in the window and stilled the flutter in my stomach, the one I still get before making a speech. It was January 2013, and this was my first one of the year. I had been invited to speak to the eleventh-grade mentees of the Step Up Women's Network, an organization in which I had been involved as a junior board member and mentor since graduating from business school.

Taking a deep breath, I rehearsed the opening lines of my speech, each word feeling suddenly inadequate. I could articulate my degrees and showcase the highlights of a résumé that glittered with success, but beneath it all, there was a tremor of something unspoken that begged for release. The conference room buzzed with the murmur of conversations and high school girl giggles. About thirty Black and brown girls from East Harlem and the Bronx sat around the conference tables that formed a U shape in the room. Their eyes, when they met mine, held a cocktail of curiosity and hesitation, a mirror of how I might have looked at that age when confronted with someone from another world.

I squared my shoulders and took a deep breath. "Good morning," I began cheerily. "I'm Daria Burke. I'm so excited to be here with you today, and to share a bit about my college and MBA studies, my career path to the beauty industry, and my current role at Estée Lauder."

I stood in a pink silk sheath and black blazer, a big black belt cinching my waist. "I remember being exactly where you are now," I continued. "Dreaming big in a world that may feel too small, wanting to create a life that your family may not understand." The words tumbled out with a mix of rehearsed and genuine enthusiasm as I talked about going away to college, then grad school, eventually recounting tales of product development days at the lab and describing the process of getting an ad into a magazine.

I scanned the room as I spoke, hopeful for engagement. Their expressions were courteous, but their body language spoke volumes—slouched shoulders of resignation, subtle eye rolls that said: "Did I really take the train to Midtown Manhattan on a Saturday morning for this?"

The silence was punctuated by a stifled yawn from a girl in a navy sweatshirt to my right. The shiny surface of my achievements seemed to glare harshly in the fluorescent light of their reality. The girls sat like statues, eyes glazed with disinterest. My words, a source of pride on the page, felt hollow and impotent in the room. I had come to inspire them, and I was falling short. A pang of understanding twisted in my gut—I was speaking at them, not to them. They needed more than the gloss of success. They needed the grit of reality, the testimony of someone who had walked in their shoes and found a way out.

"Okay," I said, my voice softer, inviting them closer. "I'm gonna go off script here for a minute." I set my notes aside, feeling a little exposed, and took a seat in the center of the room so I could be eye level with them.

"I grew up extremely poor, and I had a really difficult childhood," I began, my heart thrumming in my chest. "I was 'raised' by my mother"—I put up air quotes—"but she was lost in her own struggles, leaving me to navigate much of the world on my own."

The tone in the room shifted, became heavier, as if my words were landing in a reality that finally resonated. "I saw and experienced things no child should. I know the cold bite of winter inside a house without heat or hot water."

I confessed that my childhood had been painful and,

many times, lonely, but that I had been a strong student like they were. Then I told them how I had risen above it, stitching wings from sheer willpower and soaring across voids that once seemed impassable. And that they could do the same. I locked eyes with the girl directly in front of me, her guarded expression softening, as if my memories had unlatched something within her own. "But early on, I knew that that life wasn't mine. My life was waiting for me. And I made a promise to myself that I would find a way to it, no matter what it took."

Their faces now bore traces of interest, like shutters opening to let the light in. A few leaned forward, elbows resting on the table, eyes not leaving mine. Others exchanged glances with one another, their skepticism eroding.

"When you come from a place like that," I confessed, "I know that it can be hard to dream about success because you're so focused on survival." I let out a breath I hadn't realized I'd been holding.

"Maybe you know a version of this story." My voice was barely audible, but they heard every word. "Maybe you're sitting here today, wondering if there's a way out of your own situation. Wondering if anyone understands. I understand. I believe that everything I went through was a lesson in strength and in believing in myself. And it brought me to you."

A chorus of sniffles punctuated the silence between my words. Their hardened exteriors melted away to reveal an unguarded essence of who they were. Memories flooded back, visceral and gripping—a younger me, huddled in darkness, making silent vows to the stars that blinked coldly above the Detroit skyline.

The energy in the room shifted, a collective breath drawn in and released, leaving us all a little lighter. The girls sat up straighter, their faces mirrors of an awakening realization, reflecting a recognition of something within themselves that, perhaps, they had never dared to acknowledge. The room had come alive with something that felt like hope.

"Fifteen years ago, I was exactly where you are now. I came here to show you that what's possible for me is possible for each one of you. My story is not a fairy tale. It is far from perfect. But it is a testament to what can be made from the raw materials of hope, courage, and an unyielding belief in what can be."

During the Q&A, the girl in the navy sweatshirt whose guarded eyes had been the toughest to reach raised her hand and softly asked, "How did you not give up?"

"By realizing that giving up would mean giving in to the narrative that was written for me by circumstances, by other people's choices and mistakes."

The girls buzzed again, bees discovering a field of wildflowers after a long winter—glimmers of possibilities, of dreams unfurling their delicate wings in the warmth of newfound belief. Their eyes shone brighter, and I saw reflections of myself in them. It was as though we were all standing on the precipice of our futures together, daring to dream about what comes next.

"I want to leave you with one of my favorite quotes," I said, at last getting back to my script. "It's by Bruce Barton: 'Nothing splendid has ever been achieved, except by those who dared believe that something inside them was superior to circumstance.'" I breathed in deeply, feeling truly seen for the first time—not as the sum of my achievements, but as the culmination of everything I'd overcome to be there with them that morning.

"Thank you," I heard myself say, my heart full of gratitude "for allowing me to share my story with you. For seeing me. For letting me see you."

Their nods were slow, thoughtful, as if they were turning over my words like stones in their hands. As the last of the applause faded into a hush, I met the glances of girls who started the hour as strangers and now felt like kin.

I gathered my notes, their edges softened from anxious handling. They seemed like relics now, artifacts from a time when I believed my greatest offering lay in the tidy bullet points of a written speech rather than the raw truth of my story.

As the session concluded, three of the girls came up to me and asked if we could take a picture. One of them stayed behind.

"Your story...it's kinda like mine. And I just wanted to say thank you. For being here. And for being real with us."

Her words resonated deeper than any praise I had received before. "It's truly been my privilege," I told her.

I wanted to call Meghan. I stood outside on Sixth Avenue, letting the magnitude of the experience settle over me. My hands trembled, not from the cold, but with a kind of elation that comes from casting off shackles you've worn for so long they've become part of your skin. In that moment, I began to envision a different kind of life—one where my past and present could coexist. I had done more than show up that day; I had fully arrived.

Meghan and I hadn't spoken in nearly a year and a half since she left for LA. She was no longer my therapist, and we weren't friends. "I finally get what you meant about integration," I wanted to tell her. I imagined her blue eyes holding mine. "Today, I told my story in public for the first time and I've never felt more like myself."

Time isn't the healer we often mistake it to be. It is impartial and indifferent, an observer at best. It merely passes, unconcerned with the human condition. It is the business of living through time that does the healing—you nurse the wound and negotiate with your pain, not as an enemy but as an offering. It's in letting go of the anguish, while holding on to the wisdom it came with. There are days when the labor of this learning will overwhelm you. There will be the temptation to turn away from it, and turn back to the familiar, even if it's a prison of your own making. And in this resistance, in this instinct to fold inward, we see our self-sabotage laid bare.

In the end, the decision to turn back or to press on defines us. Audre Lorde spoke truth to such moments: "I am constantly defining my selves, for I am, as we all are, made up of so many different parts. But when those selves war within me, I am immobilized, and when they move in harmony, or allowance, I am enriched, made strong." For years, I resisted telling a version of my story that included all the parts of me. The pain of my history had left me fearful and numb, and I declared that there was no room for my past in the future I was creating. I almost missed the chance to become something more than that pain could envision for me.

"Healing from trauma is not an exorcism, it's an integration," Judith Herman famously said. It is an experience not of eradication but of reconciliation. I knew the psychic cost of cutting myself off from the past—the emotional strain, the physical toll, the spiritual disconnection. The body, with its own memory, does not forget so easily what the mind tries to bury. My vigilance was an inner war between the relentless pull of memory and my deep desire to forget. This tension eroded any sense of peace I found and left me with a soul-level exhaustion from the constant battle to segregate parts of myself.

I once floated on the surface, afraid of the depths below. The waters around me were calm, yet I knew of the undercurrents that pulled at my roots. My passage from this place of dissociation to the depths of acknowledgment began not with a plunge, but with a gentle descent, a slow immersion into the waters of my past. We do not, cannot, dissociate from the water, a substance more akin to ourselves than we might like to admit. When my feet finally touched the ocean floor, I could see that depth was not to be feared but explored. Light filtered down from above, illuminating the hidden corners of my subconscious. Facing these submerged parts of myself was like learning to breathe underwater, a practice in finding life in places I once thought uninhabitable. Mary Karr had it right when she said that no one wades deep into these waters without drowning a little. But in the surrender, you learn to float.

"It's like rinsing a sponge," Meghan once told me, referring to the ways in which integration and healing intersect. "You run it under water, squeeze, and there's more soap. So, you rinse it again and watch as the last of the soap escapes. And you think you're done." She paused, allowing the metaphor to settle before continuing. "But if you put it back under water, it turns out there's more soap there. And that's okay. It doesn't mean you've failed or that you're back at square one. It's a continuous cycle of discovery and release."

The act of healing is not a straight line. It is a series of waves, each one a lesson in balance, in the art of not tipping over. To stand upright is to move with grace, with a gentle bending of our knees. It's not a process, but a practice. It requires us to summon the willingness to take a clear, unflinching look inward, not in judgment but in wonder. To sit in stillness and look with a bravery that matches the soul's deepest cries for attention. We must learn that these emotions are as much a part of us as flesh and bone. They are the very substance from which we are made. And then, we must find the strength to take a step back and view them within the broader frame of our lives. From a distance, patterns emerge, and we can see the ways in which our past informs the present and colors the future.

Integration, then, means knitting together these detailed observations and broad understandings into a coherent sense of self. It is about acknowledging the contradictions, holding the complexities, and finding clarity in the confusion. It is a series of ongoing negotiations between the past and the present, the self and the other, the details and the bigger picture. It is delicate work, one that requires patience and the courage to face the world as it is, not as we wish it to be, and the courage to do the same with ourselves.

12

IDENTITY REPOSSESSED

D addy had a stroke." Leah's voice cut through the stillness of an ordinary afternoon the following January.

"Is he...How bad is it?" I held the phone to my ear and spoke in a voice that seemed to belong to someone else—someone who hadn't built walls around the mere mention of her parents.

"It was bad," she said, her tone tight, trembling at the edges. "He's in the ICU and he's unconscious." Stroke. ICU. I pictured a room full of machines that breathe for you when your body can't muster the strength. A pang of something—fear, or maybe sadness—fluttered momentarily, swiftly muted by years of emotional insulation.

"He's in critical condition. Are you coming back to Detroit?"

I steadied myself on the edge of the sofa.

"I don't know. I need to think about it." Familial duty

wrestled with self-preservation, an age-old conflict where there are no winners, just varying degrees of bruising.

"Okay," Leah replied after a pause, heavy with things unsaid. "Well...let me know."

"Sure," I managed before hanging up.

I paced the length of my living room, stopping in front of the window that looked out over the back garden. My reflection stared back at me, a mirror twin trapped on the other side of the glass.

"Shit," I murmured, suddenly furious, though not knowing whether my ire was over my father's condition, or over feeling like I was being pulled in.

Daddy had a stroke. I replayed her words in my mind. The man in question was, technically speaking, my father—contributor of half my genetic makeup. But he was little more than that to me. To call him my father was a statement of fact, as sterile as the word *father* itself. It lacked the intimacy and warmth of *Daddy*, or the earned respect signified by *Dad*. *Father*, to me, was devoid of the layers of love, sacrifice, and emotional investment that the other terms imply.

Would my father, I wondered, make the journey for me were our roles reversed? Would he travel six hundred miles from Detroit to be by my side? The answer came swift and unforgiving—no. As fathers go, mine had proven to be, as my mother insisted, "good for nothing." Throughout my childhood, there had been no form of child support, no cheer practice drive-bys, no threats to beat up the neighborhood bully who tormented us girls on our walks home from school, or soothing of my ego when my sophomore crush told my classmate he thought I was ugly. I allowed myself the petty luxury of cataloging the reasons why he—even potentially on his deathbed—did not warrant my presence. More than anything, he had been completely absent through every meaningful moment of my life. And anyway, what would I do with myself sitting in his hospital room? Hold vigil in silence because we shared no loving memories I could recount? What comfort could I offer a father who had given me virtually nothing but his name?

Eight years earlier, just a few months after I had first moved to New York for business school, my phone rang. An unknown number from a familiar area code interrupted my solitary walk through Washington Square Park. It was my father, whom I hadn't seen or spoken to since my freshman year of college, calling to wish me a happy birthday. I was turning twenty-six, which meant the week before, he had turned fifty-one.

"Hey Daria, it's your dad." It still strikes me that he knew to announce himself, the assumption that his voice alone wasn't enough for me to place him. "I was just calling to say happy birthday."

"Hey," I coughed up, annoyed that I had answered the call. "Thanks. Happy belated birthday to you."

"Where are you?" he asked.

"I'm in New York." His presence—even over the

phone—had a way of reducing me to the fewest possible words. My hope was that he'd get the hint that I didn't want to talk.

"New York? What you doing there?"

"I moved here for business school. I'm at NYU. I'm getting an MB—a master of business administration."

"Say what? That's my girl! I'm proud of you, Dee."

Proud of me? Suddenly, I was salivating at the chance to tell him off.

My mouth watered with rage. "You don't get to be proud of me. You aren't allowed to take pride in anything I have achieved. You did nothing to help me get to where I am. Nothing. Everything I have done, everything I am, is in spite of you."

"Daria." He tried to get a word in.

"No, let me finish. You call me out of nowhere…I don't even know the last time we spoke. You call me out of nowhere to say that you're proud of me? Don't you dare," I shouted into the phone, punctuating every word. "Don't. You. Dare. You don't deserve to be proud of me. Don't call me again. I mean it. Do not call me."

That day in Washington Square Park, I had unleashed a fury toward him, a primal and formidable anger so pure it startled even me. It was an anger born of neglect, of unmet expectations, and of the profound void that his absence had left in my life. That call, our last exchange, ended with words of such finality.

And now, after the passage of many years, he lay incapacitated, forcing me to confront my anger toward him. As I stood on the precipice of losing him forever, I found myself analyzing the nature of my intense resentment.

For days, I wavered over whether to go, ultimately choosing to stay in New York. The decision not to go to him was not born of apathy but of a profound acknowledgment of our estrangement. In the aftermath of my choice, I stumbled into a truth, stark and undeniable. My anger had quietly confessed its true identity; it was not merely the product of my father's neglect or the embodiment of abandonment. It was grief impersonating fury, a mourning for the connection that remained only a notion in our shared history.

I also thought ahead to whether, if the stroke did prove fatal, I would attend his funeral. It would be an opportunity to say goodbye, I reasoned, not just to him, but to the version of myself that had remained trapped in this bitterness. But did I need him to die to do that? I didn't need there to be a funeral to lay to rest the anger and sadness I carried my entire life. He lived, but I decided that when the time did come, I would attend his funeral, and I would do it with a clear heart.

Many years later, I would also learn that the doctors had found heroin in his system when he suffered the stroke. I felt further justified for making the call not to go to Detroit but I no longer allowed his failings as a father to dictate the terms of my compassion toward him as person.

As my father's health threatened to disrupt my life, I had been contemplating my own unraveling. After eight years in New York, I was tired. I was thirty-three, already burned out, worn down by the constant chase. I blamed it on New York's ceaseless pace, rather than on my self-imposed, insatiable appetite to achieve. The city had not demanded my allegiance to this frenetic pace; I had volunteered it.

While at Estée Lauder, it dawned on me that I knew many mid-career Black women, myself included, who found themselves with fewer mentors and less community as they became more senior in their organizations. In response, I founded an organization called Black MBA Women. My initial thought was simply "We should all know each other," so I created a LinkedIn group and invited the women I knew. A few weeks after starting the group, I hosted our first happy hour and more than forty of our sixty or so members came out, including one woman who had driven up from Philadelphia. I was stunned. Within a year, the group grew to nearly five hundred women, and by January 2014, it had doubled in size and included members from outside of the United States.

The founding of Black MBA Women earned me invitations to speak at conferences and lead career workshops all over the country and to write for publications like *Black Enterprise* and the *Huffington Post*. My work was highlighted in national media, and I was able to secure corporate sponsors to host events featuring high-profile women authors and

C-level executives. I never had a plan for how to grow or nurture what I had built; I just knew that I wanted to do something of consequence, to stand at the center of something meaningful. Eventually, even Black MBA Women would not be enough to satisfy my appetite for more. No matter how fast I ran, satisfaction remained stubbornly ahead, an ever-moving target. Each achievement, rather than providing relief, only inflamed the condition further. It was an endless climb up the mountain without ever stopping to look at the view. Every two or three years, I'd get the itch to trade up for a bigger title, higher salary, more responsibility. It was time for another move.

Around the time of my father's stroke, a business school colleague introduced me to a recruiter for a major national PR agency that was looking to add beauty and personal care to its portfolio and wanted to hire an industry insider. I began interviewing for the role, and things moved quickly—a call with an internal recruiting manager was followed by a day trip to Chicago for a marathon of meetings with six different people. I got their offer while in the car before I'd even made it to O'Hare to fly back to New York. Within days, I reviewed, negotiated, and accepted the offer, excited by the promise of a new start in a new city where my dreams could find their footing.

Movers would soon arrive to pack up my New York apartment and haul everything off to Chicago, where it would go into storage while I lived in corporate housing and looked for a permanent place to live. Several friends threw me a fabulous going-away party at a champagne bar in Tribeca and a crowd came to send me off; they'd even made a scrapbook that people signed with sweet expressions of friendship and goodwill. That was the first time I would question whether I was making the right decision. But I told myself that it was just premature homesickness. Not every day in New York was full of the kind of affection that one finds only at going-away parties.

Two days before my departure, I got a call from a producer on the *Melissa Harris-Perry* show on MSNBC. She had received my name from a mutual acquaintance who also worked on the show. They were planning a segment on Lean In's "Ban Bossiness" campaign, and how we speak to women in politics more broadly, and they wanted me to join as a guest. The segment would air live on the morning of Saturday, March 22, just hours before I was scheduled to fly to Chicago. A black town car picked me up and escorted me to 30 Rock. I arrived dressed for my appearance and headed into hair and makeup and got mic'ed for the segment, hosted by Jonathan Capehart, who guest-hosted for Melissa Harris-Perry during her maternity leave.

I had been live on air before—on the *Today* show, where I first appeared as a "model" for a Rent the Runway segment in which nearly all of the company's female employees at the time wore dresses from the site. The second time I would appear in a disaster of a segment that was a follow-up to a

Lucky magazine feature I'd been in. The styling, hair, and makeup had all been quite tragic, and I'd thought I looked "huge" on camera. But this experience was different, a dream come true, really: my national television debut as "Daria Burke" would have me speaking about an area of passion— girls and women in leadership—on my favorite talk show.

Somehow, the two-minute segment both flew by and stretched on forever. I loved every second of the experience: the producer in my ear counting down to when we were live, sitting at the desk across from Jonathan Capehart, with the other esteemed guests. I got the same rush of exhilaration I'd felt when I performed onstage during college. When the segment ended, adrenaline was still flooding my system. I was leaving *this*? I imagined the possibility of a new career trajectory, one that could veer into both media and advocacy work. Yet, Chicago awaited—a commitment made, a path chosen.

"Great job today," a producer offered, snapping me back to reality. "You should consider doing this more often."

"Thank you so much," I beamed. The compliment ricocheted inside me as I headed into the elevator and down to the car waiting to take me to the airport. I felt the weight of my decision in each step.

Once in Chicago, I embraced the move and new role with the exuberance of someone who needed its promise to be true. The PR firm greeted me with open arms; I was the fresh blood from New York, there to invigorate and innovate.

I threw myself into the work and for a time, it seemed as though I'd found my footing on unfamiliar ground.

Then, without warning, the foundation cracked.

Four months into my new job, I was let go. I had been managing a client that was a terrible fit for my experience and their needs while trying to help win new business when the company lost a big client and millions in fees in my practice. I wasn't fully billable yet, and was, therefore, expensive. I had been waiting to be restaffed. Instead, I lost my job. Last in, first out. They gave me two weeks' severance and that was it.

Losing my job was a crushing blow, causing me to question everything I had once felt so sure of. The life and career I had worked so hard to build suddenly seemed incredibly fragile. Was this life that I had built for myself real if my success could be erased so easily? Could it be that I—the careful, cautious, A student, always concerned with the consequences of my actions—was in fact impulsive and reckless, just one bad career decision away from ruining my entire life? I'd spent years doing everything I could to avoid becoming like my mother, punishing myself for any shadow of similarity that I detected. But now I wondered, was I, deep down, more like my mother than I cared to admit?

I lived in fear of messing up, even if there wasn't anyone to disappoint other than myself. I had spent most of my life on the hedonic treadmill, much like an addict chasing that next fix, my pursuit of success a compulsion, a need that dominated all else in my life. The adrenaline rush of my next accomplishment, each feat a fleeting high that dissipated as quickly as it arrived, left behind an ever-growing hunger for more.

Dopamine, a cunning alchemist of the brain, transformed my ambition into a visceral craving. Each accomplishment triggers its release, a flood that washes over the brain, bathing it in a glow of pleasure, a reward for the deed done. Soon, the glow fades, leaving an empty space that demands to be filled again. Do it too many times and your tolerance increases. The brain, now accustomed to these surges of dopamine, craves the rush, rewiring itself in pursuit of the high. It adapts to anything that affects its function: cocaine, alcohol, sugar, sex, shopping, scrolling, success. The cycle perpetuates—a task of endless pursuit, where satisfaction is always just beyond the grasp, and the next peak looms, always a bit higher than the last. With each cycle, the toll becomes more evident, not just in the mind, but in the body. In responding to the brain's demands, it readies itself for the next chase, muscles tensed, heart rate elevated, all systems go. My ambitions had become my masters, their orders etched in the stone of "more" and "next," in the relentless ticking of my schedule. The goals I served so devoutly kept me in a constant state of striving, a willing captive to a standard of excellence that had no limits. My unwavering loyalty a misplaced devotion that cost more than it would ever reward.

Having lost my job, I felt a deep sense of shame, and my first instinct was to withdraw and hide the news. Instead, I texted two of my girlfriends letting them know what had happened. I wasn't ready to talk, but I knew better than to keep it to myself. Despair may be contagious, but depression thrives in isolation. A third friend immediately sent me money, nearly enough to pay my rent for a month, no questions asked. Another reached out to me every day to make sure I was okay.

I took walks on the lake. I got rest. I kept my hair appointment. I made space for being.

A few days later, I reached out to my friend Mark to share the news. Even when he drives me crazy, he never fails to make me laugh and make everything feel better.

"Wow! You just started," he said. "That's terrible." My normally chatty friend was at a loss for words.

"That's an understatement," I said, dreading the number of times I would have to have a version of this conversation. "I feel like the universe is telling me I made a mistake."

"Okay. Well, time for a classic Daria rebound," he said with supreme confidence.

"I don't know if I have it in me," I confessed.

"Yeah, you do," Mark reassured me in the matter-of-fact way he says everything. "You have been through so much worse. The loss in that group has nothing to do with you. It wasn't even your client."

He was right. But I couldn't get over the fact that I had

failed to do my due diligence on the financial health of the firm, a mistake I attributed to nothing but my own blinding ambition. I now saw this as a lapse that had cost me not only my job but also my sense of self. My identity and self-worth were so rooted in things that other people could measure, things outside of myself. I believed that losing my job was proof that I hadn't been worthy of the good things people thought about me.

The day after my conversation with Mark, I woke up and actually felt...okay. For the first time since I was a little girl, younger than my memory will allow, I felt like I had family. I did not realize how long I'd been going, how hard I had been pushing, how exhausted I was, until my friends stood behind me, and caught me when I fell. This was what it feels like to be held.

Earlier in the summer, I had planned a week-long trip to Martha's Vineyard with two big groups of friends. I felt guilty at the idea of going when I should have been job-hunting but decided that being surrounded by friends was exactly what I needed. I had made many a solitary pilgrimage on my survivor's journey. I would no longer choose to go it alone. I had spent so many years avoiding being seen, for fear that my vulnerabilities were weaknesses to be used against me. Hiding kept me safe from judgment and criticism, and from love.

I packed for the week and flew to New York. My friend Tracey had borrowed her dad's SUV so she, her then boyfriend, now husband, John, and I could fill it with our excess of luggage, beach essentials, and snacks. We loaded everything the next morning and made the four-hour drive from New York City to Woods Hole, where we could drive onto the ferry that would take us, and the car, to Martha's Vineyard.

As the ferry pulled away from the dock, the sea breeze tangled my hair, carrying away some of the heaviness that had been pressing down on me. I watched the island grow, feeling the nourishing magic of the Vineyard drawing near. I wanted to take it all in, but a voice over the loudspeaker interrupted my daydream.

"Please return to your vehicles. We're approaching the terminal."

Ask anyone who has spent time on Martha's Vineyard why they love it, and they'll likely mention the sense of community. But it was more than that. Stepping onto the island, I was greeted by something that felt familial, ancestral even. There was a sacredness to it, as if the island's natural beauty had been enhanced by its cultural legacy.

I was in a seven-bedroom shared house on the shoreline of the historically Black Inkwell Beach in Oak Bluffs with thirteen other people, while Tracey and John stayed with two other couples in quaint and less-trafficked Edgartown, but we'd see each other throughout the week for lunches and sunsets and game nights at one another's houses.

That time on the Vineyard turned out to be healing in a way that I couldn't have imagined. I woke to the smell and sight of the ocean, my heart rate steadied, my mind lulled into a semi-meditative state called drifting, where we are engaged with the world around us without any focus on achievement. We made meals in groups; the women would cook breakfast one day and the men made dinner. I spent my mornings walking or running on the beach, the sun warming my skin. We played card and board games, and spent afternoons in town getting lunch, ice cream, and swag from the Black Dog. We rode mopeds to the other towns and went to a clambake on the beach. We chatted with locals and other vacationers like old friends. In the evenings, we gathered on the wraparound porch after dinner and shared stories, dreams, and fears. Each day my heart lightened by the love and laughter of friends old and new.

Confiding in my friends, I allowed the dam of my vulnerability to break, and in their embrace, I met the full strength of the community I had built. *This* was my safety net. Their counsel was a unanimous chorus calling me back to New York City. Yet the reality of my circumstances—locked into a luxury rental on Lake Shore Drive with a modest and dwindling savings account and without suitable job prospects in Chicago—left me with very few choices. The solution, as unorthodox as it seemed, was born of desperation.

A few weeks later, I sublet my Chicago apartment and ventured to Brooklyn, into the cramped yet comforting confines of a three-bedroom Park Slope apartment that Nicky shared with her boyfriend, now husband, Jenny, and his roommate, Dean. The presence of Ewing, Jenny's

170-pound English mastiff—when paired with my Cavalier King Charles spaniel, Gatsby—added to the chaos and contentment. Imagine, if you will, four thirtysomething adults (a Jamaican, a Haitian, an Englishman, and an American) in three bedrooms with two dogs and one bathroom in a Brooklyn brownstone. It's the stuff of network sitcoms.

It was there, amid the clutter of shared lives and the negotiation of communal living, that I encountered my own unraveling. I had reached what I could only describe then as rock bottom, a term that felt both clichéd and acutely precise in its depiction of my state. Other than Gatsby and the two suitcases I'd brought with me, nothing there was mine.

In those first days, I couldn't shake the feeling that needing more somehow made me less worthy. When Nicky let me cram my things into her already-full closets and she carved out a corner of the medicine cabinet, so that I didn't have to carry my toiletries to the bathroom co-ed style in a shower caddy, I felt an uncomfortable sense of intrusion. I didn't want to be a burden on Nicky and Jenny. My being there was clearly disrupting their lives. But they didn't treat me as a burden; they saw me as family. Nicky refused any money I offered to offset the cost of my being there, and they were always so gracious when I restocked the fridge or came home with candles or bottles of wine. Despite my reluctance to get too comfortable, the apartment became a sanctuary. We threw house parties and watched TV together as a household. We took care of each other's dogs, and Jenny, the best cook I know, taught me how to make pernil and ropa vieja. They helped stitch me back together.

It was there, in that state of forced humility, that I was compelled to confront another uncomfortable truth: I had been living on borrowed equity. So much of my identity had been outsourced, built on a foundation of external achievements that were as fleeting as they were superficial, linked to assets I didn't actually own but had been temporarily granted access to. It was the applause at the end of a speech, the prestige of my alma maters, the job titles that elicited nods of approval, the salary band that placed me within a certain socioeconomic stratum, and the tangible outputs I could produce for others—these had been the metrics by which I had measured my worth.

In carving a way out of Detroit, I had become complicit in my own subjugation to a set of societal norms—dreams even—that I wasn't even sure belonged to me. Now, stripped of it all, the scaffolding had collapsed. There was nowhere to hide. I was adrift, confronted with the daunting question of who I was without an important title and the world's approval to define it for me.

This rock bottom would be more than a low point. It would be the foundation upon which I could rebuild, starting with what I call an owned identity. Unlike borrowed equity, owned identity is an intrinsic value and self-perception rooted within, independent of external achievements or recognition. A sense of self built on personal values, inner strengths, passions, and the unique qualities that make a person who they are. This identity emerges from an internal process, one rooted in self-cultivation, untouched by things and people outside of ourselves. It can be neither given nor taken away and is resilient to the ebb and flow of social acceptance.

For months, I hid out in Brooklyn. Aside from my close friends, no one knew that I'd moved back to New York. I was ashamed to have boomeranged back so soon after leaving for Chicago and to be living out of suitcases in a friend's spare bedroom. I felt like a coward for hiding but needed the time away to connect with my own feelings about my situation. Mark was right—I had survived the worst thing that would ever happen to me. I was being set up for a rebound, but it wouldn't be in the style of "classic Daria." None of my child-hood survival tools had utility here. It was time for a differ-ent approach.

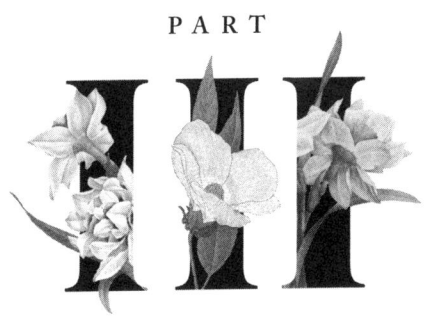
RECLAMATION

To accept one's past—one's history—is not the same thing as drowning in it; it is learning how to use it. An invented past can never be used; it cracks and crumbles under the pressures of life like clay in a season of drought.

—James Baldwin

13

SWEET SURRENDER

After a three-month job search in New York City and nearly six months with Nicky and Jenny, I got a call from a recruiter about a role that would leverage my prestige beauty experience. It was a newly created role on the retail strategy team at CVS Health, which then ranked number seven on the Fortune 500. The recruiter talked about the company's increased commitment to its health mission as evidenced in its decision to stop selling tobacco products, and its desire to demonstrate its healthy equity and authority in the retail store by prioritizing "healthy" beauty and personal care.

As head of Beauty Growth Strategy & Innovation at CVS, I would be working from their corporate headquarters in Woonsocket, Rhode Island, about fifteen minutes north of Providence. Having spent nearly a decade in New York working for the world's biggest beauty brands, I struggled to picture myself in the sterile, suburban offices of a health-care company in the smallest state with the longest name. The population of the Upper West Side of Manhattan is bigger than all of Providence, a fact I would cite to friends in a plea for their understanding of my disenchantment with the idea. The role itself was a great opportunity, however, and I needed a job, so I reluctantly packed my company-rented SUV and began the four-hour drive to New England.

An hour outside of Providence on I-95, the word suddenly descended upon me with newfound purpose, flashing like ticker tape across my windshield—Providence: *a manifestation of divine care and direction; timely preparation for future eventualities.* Not once in the six-week interview process had the meaning of the city's name dawned on me, but now the message was crystal clear. It wasn't about the job. I was being steered toward something greater, barreling toward a destiny named after divine intervention. The irony was rich enough to draw a laugh.

"Okay," I said with a smile, taking both hands off the wheel and raising them in the air, a submission to my own transformation.

Every loss I'd suffered up to this point became an invitation to release what was holding me back, and to declare—awakened and with intention—who I wanted to be: the protagonist of a conscious and curious life. As I drove, I felt myself letting go of the ideas I had about exactly what my journey would be like, the heavy, worn-out attachments I had forged from my fears and failings, the desperate need to manipulate my self-image and dictate every outcome. How my life felt was suddenly far more important than how it appeared. The road stretched on, an invitation to the unknown, and I pressed the accelerator just a bit more firmly, eager to answer the call.

The destination mattered less than the journey now. Providence emerged on the horizon like a promise of beginning, of becoming, of belonging—to myself. A promise not of a place, but of a path toward wholeness. The city had lent its name not as a marker of my arrival, but as a symbol of my willingness to journey—to embrace the known and the unknown—undertaken with acceptance and free of resentment.

"Time to let go," I said, my voice steady but grounded by the gravity of what I was leaving behind. I could feel a chapter of my life close with a gentle click.

In the months that followed, I immersed myself in the work at CVS, channeling my newfound perspective into tangible outcomes. The job, once a reluctant compromise, had begun to blossom into a field of opportunity. I was doing strategic work that was fulfilling enough, and I worked with really smart people whom I liked a great deal. I had even opened up to several of them, a first for me. I spent the summer exploring more of Martha's Vineyard and visiting Newport and Cape Cod. The charm of Providence had grown on me ("It's a good food town," I'd say with confidence), and New York City was only a three-hour train ride away.

As my thirty-fifth birthday approached, I found myself reflecting on the journey that had led me there. The move to Providence had been a leap of faith and a lifeline in a dark time. I wanted to mark the milestone not just as a celebration of age, but as an homage to the journey itself. East Hampton called to me, not just for its serene beauty and the quiet luxury it offered, but for what it represented—a place where I could pause and honor the path and the people that had brought me to that moment.

We'd spent a small fortune for the rental and braved rain that came at us sideways, just to spend time together. But then, that friend brought weed into the house, and I let some invisible hand pull me out of what had been a perfectly lovely weekend.

In those early hours the next morning, as the house began to stir with the first sounds of waking life, I lay in bed trying to contend with what had happened. Part of me longed to keep my eyes closed, to resist the intrusion of daylight and the certainty it would bring. I was afraid to open my eyes and acknowledge that waking up meant facing reality, of being aware and accepting the responsibility of healing myself. You can't sleepwalk your way to healing. I feared that in seeing clearly, I would be asked to let go.

Ultimately, I wrote it off as a weird night and a very specific, isolated incident. I wanted to move on. It would take me years to see how the night of my birthday dinner had been the start of something giving way. But the echoes of that evening clung to me like a second skin the entire drive back to Providence—my friend's tone-deaf behavior, her disregard for my discomfort, my startling visceral reaction. This had been no mere overindulgence in wine or even the unexpected presence of an unwelcome substance. It was a reckoning with a past that had sat, silent and brooding, waiting for a moment to step forward into the light. The act of purchasing *Triggers* by Marshall Goldsmith a month after that night had not struck me as significant at the time. It was a decision made almost on autopilot, a title picked from a shelf in a moment of idle curiosity. Now the book seems less like a choice and more like a gentle nudge from the universe.

Triggers are not merely psychological land mines; they are the keys to the locked doors of our most formative experiences. In the wake of my thirty-fifth birthday, I began to see them with new clarity. Our environments are filled with these stimuli—seemingly benign yet capable of unsettling our present with echoes of the past. I understood this on some level; it was why I left Detroit, why I spent as little time there as possible. Even as a teenager, I knew I couldn't grow there, couldn't fulfill my potential in an environment that dug at old wounds and stifled new beginnings.

For years, I charted the course of my healing by the absence of triggers in my life. But there were, in the subtle manifestations of anxiety, activations that elicited a knee-jerk response. A trigger won't always present itself with a big flashing light that says, "Look here!" Most don't. They never come as a warning or when there's any real danger. Tell me that my house is about to catch fire, my close friend needs emergency surgery, that democracy as we know it is over, and I won't feel triggered. They come instead when I am steeped in the small acts of everyday interactions, while watching a mother-daughter moment in a movie, when someone cuts me off while I'm speaking and I feel ignored or disregarded, when I'm pressured to have an answer for something that I need time to consider, or when I find a small leak in the basement at the end of a stressful week.

In the earliest hours of the morning, I began to wake up and sit in stillness. Before getting out of bed, I would declare my intentions for the day, visualizing the energy I would need to summon to move toward them. These intentions started off small, and I would write them down. I would call in patience, or endurance if I had a big day of meetings.

Something began working on me, in me. Meditation became a way of climbing back into myself. I began to practice connected detachment, a means of engaging with the world with empathy and compassion while maintaining an inner distance to protect my peace. In this, I am connected to the feelings, the people, the task, but detached from the outcome. In this mastery of my inner authority, I began to develop a greater emotional independence from the external world and to pay attention to the subtle shifts and the quiet undercurrents that influence my state of being. I notice what

I am noticing. I find clarity. I am discerning. I know what to look for, what to let go of and when.

When my ego becomes inflated and I catch myself searching for scraps of superiority to cover up all the ways I've undervalued myself, I know that something has threatened my sense of self-worth. *I'm not comfortable here.* Whenever frustration arises, I am probably forcing something that isn't happening with ease. *This isn't fair; when is it my turn?* It's in the moment of pause before I respond that I find the clarity to choose a different path.

Life, at its core, is a series of choices made in the shadows before the light. I decided then that my choices would be acts of intention, each day unfolding in a series of conscious moments like pearls on a string. I slowly became more present, more engaged with the world around me in a way that was both open and protective.

If that night in East Hampton was a nudge, finding the photo of Grandma's accident two years later was like being shoved over the cliff's edge into a free fall. Such an awakening, I have since discovered—the tear in the veil of illusion we wrap around our lives—generally comes in a way that we cannot ignore.

"Trauma comes back as a reaction, not a memory," Bessel van der Kolk says.

It was as if I had been walking through a landscape of myth and memory, suddenly thrust into a clearing I had forgotten, forced to acknowledge the layers of loss that had sedimented over time. The act of repeatedly facing my emotions had cultivated a capacity to deal with more, like watching scenes with the shutter of a camera lens until I could open the aperture and see more. Each tear shed, each moment of despair confronted, was a step toward a spring of my own making—a season of growth watered by the very emotions I once feared would drown me. As I became more adept at surviving my emotions, the subconscious protections around my hidden traumas began to loosen and I found the strength that I couldn't access in my suffering.

Memories and events like my grandmother's death, encapsulated in physical sensations or reactions, may remain dormant until an external prompt—a gesture or a photograph—brings them to the surface. Somatic memories are etched within like ancient carvings on a weathered stone. They speak of loss and love, of pain so profound it can only be expressed through the body's own language. What we bury has a way of resurfacing, eager to reclaim its rightful space in our lives. Some of us suddenly get sick for no obvious reason, some of us can't fall or stay asleep, some of us struggle to find joy even when it's dancing right in front of us. The process of healing involves not only the mind's reconciliation with the past but also the body's. These memories, locked away in muscle and marrow, held the key to understanding the language of my past, a dialect of emotions that gave voice to the unspeakable.

And so it came to pass that the discovery of a photograph—a relic of my grandmother's tragic departure from this world—summoned what had once been hidden in the shadows of my subconscious into something urgent and unavoidable.

14

HIDDEN GEMS

I am out with lanterns,
looking for myself.

—Emily Dickinson

By the time I bought my house in the fall of 2018, I had spent nearly a year arming myself with knowledge of neuroplasticity and epigenetics, early childhood brain development, and ACE scores. Facts and figures became my weapons, a buffer between myself and the messy reality of being touched by living. My healing, too, had largely been an intellectual pursuit, a study in the theoretical, a dispassionate study of myself. I dug as deep as I could, but I still could not get directly to *it*.

Trauma doesn't live in the bright light of intellect. It lurks in the subconscious realms where we store fragments of memory and emotion from times before we had the words to name them, dwelling in places reason cannot reach. The etymology of *psychology* hints at this, with *psyche* meaning "soul"—a reminder of the profound connection between our inner worlds and the disciplines that seek to understand them. True insight and growth, therefore, reside in the silent conversations between our conscious intentions and subconscious beliefs.

On the day of my home inspection, I noticed that the seams along the vaulted ceilings were cracked. I pulled the inspector aside. "Is that cause for concern?" I asked, looking up to direct his attention. "Does this suggest that there may be an issue with the roof?"

"Nah. It's totally normal. Happens all the time," he assured me, and went on to explain. "What happens is, the rafters move around as the seasons change. Wood expands and contracts. You want 'em to have room to move around a bit so that a strong wind doesn't just lift the roof off the house." I thought of Dorothy and Toto in the house when the cyclone carried it away.

"When the rafters move," he continued, "the drywall moves with the framing and if it moves enough, the drywall splits, nails pop, what have you. I been a contractor for thirty years and it happens in my house too. Finally got tired of fixin' it and put beams up to cover it. But your roof? It's good."

"I see. So my options are either to live with it or cover it up?" I felt relieved to know the issue was cosmetic but underwhelmed by the solutions.

"Basically, yeah," he said with a kind of finality. "Unless

you want to completely redo the framing and put up a whole new roof."

In six years of owning my house, I have fixed the cracks once. I don't notice them any less, but I have learned to live with them. I understand why they're there. Each new crack reminds me of what trust is.

For twenty years, I moved through life—a transient existence marked by dorm rooms, summer sublets, and rentals spanning Ann Arbor, Houston, DC, New York City, Chicago, Providence, and back to New York City. Each move ended with me handing over my only set of keys to a landlord, leaving me empty-handed, without a place to truly call my own. During my eight-month house hunt, I bought a charming set of keychains: two solid brass bars, one engraved with *Town*, the other with *Country*. Each had its own ring, representing two homes. For the first time in two decades, I would have two sets of house keys, one of which I would never have to return. The home I had hoped for had become real.

The day I closed on my house felt like a monumental shift. It was a Friday, and I decided to stay there for the weekend. I didn't care that it would be empty. I needed to be there. After the closing, I picked up a sandwich from Citarella and headed up toward Gardiner's Bay, my rental car loaded with the essentials: an air mattress, a laundry basket packed with a set of sheets, towels, and a blanket, rolls of toilet paper and paper towels, my vintage Louis Vuitton duffel with clothes for two days, and my laptop. I barely had a cell signal, but internet service and a security system were scheduled to be installed the next day.

I pulled into the driveway, the gravel crunching beneath the tires. It sounded like the beach. I parked and just sat there, staring at the house and the grounds, somewhat stupefied by what I had just done. I took inventory of each tree and shrub on the property—the lone magnolia that stood along the brick path leading up to the porch, the lavender tree straddling my bedroom and living room windows, the crape myrtle clustered on the side of the house, the row of rhododendrons. And then there were the pines and oaks so tall that they appeared to be the overseers of the land. I imagine they were there to watch the house be built.

Getting out of the car, I felt a mix of pride and disbelief as I turned my back to the house and took a couple of pictures of myself with it in the background. Standing on the porch, I found the key to the front door. I swung the door open and stepped over the threshold into the house. The air inside was cool and still, the silence of a space waiting to be filled with life.

As furniture arrived and I filled the closets and cabinets and drawers with things that I would need for weekend and, eventually, longer stays, I found myself soon being able to drive out to the house from my apartment without packing a bag. For the first time, I was not a guest in my own life; I was home. One Sunday morning, during my routine of putting everything away, I went to place my laundry basket in the bedroom closet. Suddenly, it dawned on me: "I have a linen closet." After decades of living in one-bedroom apartments, I had brought the same way of living and functioning to this new environment. My house was teaching me to expand, to take up more space.

"We all walk in shoes too small for us," Carl Jung said, hinting at the ways we limit ourselves. Where had I been playing small? I asked this aloud, opened my journal, and decided to make a list. As my fingers brushed the page, I considered the roles handed down to me—the responsible one, the superstar performer who was seen and not heard—each carrying its own implicit message. I jotted down what came to mind: *Be good. Be useful. Be invisible. Don't ask for anything. Don't make trouble.* "Speaking up" meant "talking back," and so, as a child, my voice retreated until it was a mere whisper, lost in a world that demanded compliance. How could I be expected to honor my voice as an adult when every attempt to do so throughout my life had been met with punishment?

"I hope you grow out of this silly phase," my mother would say, her words echoing in my mind. I wrote them down too. She said this in annoyance whenever I got too exuberant as a child. She only encouraged my playful spirit when it pleased her, discouraging anything she deemed as attention-seeking. I imagine that this was why I'd felt drawn to dance and theater as a teenager and young adult. Performing had been a way to express myself without boundaries imposed on me.

I could put everything into the character I was playing and leave it all on the stage. No one would judge me for that.

I continued writing, putting to paper the beliefs that I had internalized. My mother often told me that I was a headache—a pounding reminder of another mouth to feed, another body to clothe, another soul to shepherd through the mess of life when she could barely tend to her own. She seemed to resent my sensitive nature, hating that it manifested as tears that needed wiping, feelings that required suppressing. I learned to bury my compassion beneath a layer of stoicism, though deep down I remained that same sensitive soul, wary of revealing too much. I was also taught that being too nice made me weak. When it came to the outside world, it was better to be a bitch than a pushover.

As I wrote, I reflected on the shame I'd felt over not being properly cared for as a child, and how this shame had stayed with me in my adult life. This neglect wasn't just the absence of care—it was the presence of a pervasive belief that I was unworthy of it. Uncelebrated birthdays reinforced my insignificance. Missed school events signaled I didn't matter. Nights when my sister and I had to figure out our own dinner and put ourselves to bed were a reminder of how easily I could be forgotten. I felt shame for craving love and connection, the lie being that I shouldn't need so much and what I did need, I should have been able to give myself. For lacking happy childhood memories. For the ways in which my naivete about the world allowed me to be taken advantage of.

For feeling untethered without family stories or traditions or an obvious place to go for Christmas. I felt shame that all of this still made me sad.

And this shame had driven me to spend much of my life working to justify my existence in the world. It left me hustling for my worth at work, choosing boyfriends and bosses who were less than I deserved. I played small every time I stayed too long in the wrong job or relationship or clung to an identity I'd outgrown. I played small every time I said "yes" without stopping to ask myself whether what was being asked of me was what I even wanted. I hid my true self every time I silenced my wanting, opting instead for the kind of overindulging that left me feeling hollow and ashamed. My cravings for more—more love, more understanding, more of a fully expressed life—had been dammed up until they burst forth in binges that only deepened my hunger. I hadn't allowed myself to want more than was deemed acceptable. I'd repressed the instinct to fully devour my dreams, refusing my ravenous appetite for wonder and wandering. To let desire be my teacher, to listen deeply and courageously to its lessons, which were taught in the language of longing.

As brave as I had been, I had also lived a life dictated by fear and sensibility. *Don't fuck this up, D.B.* The decisions I made were driven by what was acceptable to want. As a girl, I'd colored within the lines, and I was praised for doing so. Playing by the rules was the only way to guarantee security and my way out of Detroit. The advice I received was often laced with practicality—from where I went to college and what kind of graduate degree to pursue, to the interests I allowed myself to explore. I became boring trying to be good. I had pledged a lukewarm loyalty to a life that made sense, a devotion that manifested in living the kind of life that no one would care to write stories about.

I thought of the roles we inherit and unknowingly inhabit. Messages that make certain parts of ourselves feel unsafe. A single story can evolve into a trait. (Daria is the smart one. Leah is the pretty one.) Multiple narratives metastasize into an identity. (Poverty is proof of one's failure.) Everything else goes into the shadow, a term Swiss psychiatrist Carl Jung gave to the underside of our conscious selves—the hidden, the repressed, the parts we abandoned in childhood's complex negotiations, the repository for all we have disowned, denied, and deemed unworthy of the light. The shadow is where we hide the raw, unscripted facets of our personalities out of fear of shame or rejection because they did not align with the image of the "ideal" self.

"Everyone carries a shadow, and the less it is embodied in the individual's conscious life, the blacker and denser it is," Jung wrote. There reside two selves within each of us—one that we revere and one that we forsake. Fragments of ourselves that we feel compelled to discard in fact reveal what we must reclaim. These aspects of ourselves demand recognition and must be knitted back into our conscious existence. When they remain unexplored, our personalities suffer an impoverishment, a kind of spiritual malnutrition, where, disembodied, these traits wither in the harsh light of our disregard.

The problem with leaving it unconscious is akin to living in a house divided. My own shadow, a ghost of my creation, loomed large and distorted, both reflection and caricature. I had little tolerance for deeply broken people, a reaction to the wounds in others that love was working to heal in me. I began to tally the accumulation of everything I had pushed away, making an enemy of every part of myself unworthy of the persona I presented to the world. I believe the feelings I had about losing Grandma lived there too. Somewhere deep down, I must have feared that allowing myself access to the pain of her death and everything that came with it would leave me in the same condition as my mother. And when I did finally begin to unfasten all that had unfolded, I intellectualized it and did as much as I could to avoid feeling it.

That is, until I allowed my heart to break for everything that had happened to me since Grandma died. That article had been the first tangible proof I'd seen of the event that caused our lives to unravel, and it embodied all that I had lost. Aside from a few photos of photos that my cousin, Nikki, has sent me after going through random boxes in Uncle Frank's basement, I have no physical evidence of my childhood. There are no baby pictures of me and Mom, or of the two of us and Leah. There is not a single picture from my fourth birthday party, the one where Markie, the boy next door, blew out the candles on my cake before I could. There is no trace of the white angora sweater that Grandma bought me. I remember crying when it no longer fit. None of my report cards or geometry trophies. No cheer uniform or varsity jacket. No prom dress or yearbooks. There is nothing left.

I had spent thirty years holding a broken heart. It was there, cocooned in my own hard-earned serenity, that I finally felt safe enough to travel to my interior home. To visit every location that was unknown, tour all the rooms closed off behind locked doors, reclaim every site that had been neglected, declare them all as landmarks for myself. My shadow, the host of my darkest dreams, was no longer content to be sidelined. And it stipulated a different strategy, not silencing but engaging in a dialogue. This dialogue with my shadow couldn't be a one-sided look at my behavior or the things that had happened to me; it had to be an honest conversation with the side of myself that I had for so long denied. It wasn't enough to acknowledge her existence. I had to learn her language, sit with her, and by some alchemy, turn my betrayal into acceptance. This acceptance would not come easily. It would require a steadfast and ongoing commitment to be in dialogue with the unseen, to sit with ambiguity, until I was able to endure the discomfort of growth. To find salvation, in the realization that I am capable of returning to my inner child and picking up where my parents left off.

My first attempt at an active meditation for shadow work

was awkward, like walking into a blind date not knowing who is going to show up and what mood they will be in.

"Are you ready for this?" I dared my reflection in the mirror the first time I tried the visualization, meeting the gaze of a woman who knew the cost of looking inward. But I couldn't help but smile. There was humor, too, in the absurdity of the human condition—the lengths we go to avoid the very things that could set us free. *What stands in the way becomes the way.*

I sat quietly on the sofa, the hum of the world fading as I closed my eyes. My surroundings dissolved, and I found myself transported to a solitary stretch of beach. I walked barefoot along the shoreline, feeling the warmth of the sun cover me. In the distance I saw her, my nine-year-old self, deeply engrossed in the business of building a small fortress in the sand with careful hands.

Approaching her felt like crossing a bridge between worlds. I knelt beside her, feeling again the smallness that once defined me, the enormity of the world pressing close. "Hello, little one," I began, my voice soft but sure. "I am the 'you' that is yet to come. I have traveled paths you will dream of and ones you can't yet imagine. I am here to be with you, to show you that you're safe and to tell you that you are loved. I know things are hard now, but I promise you they get better. You already have everything you need."

I took her small, sandy hand in mine, feeling the pulse of our shared heartbeat. I revealed to her what lay ahead—of the strength that would rise from our challenges, the sweetness that would follow the bitter.

"I am always with you," I promised. "You will never be without my love."

Returning to the stillness of my house, tears cascaded freely, a release as much as a relief. The meditation had become a healing passage, a channel through which I return to her, to us, as needed.

This ritual also helped me see the starkness of my inner child's perspective—how the absence of maternal care had been internalized as a measure of my own value, how a home fraught with peril had tinted my view of the world and my place in it. It was my sacred task to console this little girl, to affirm that she was—that we were—secure now. Not to fear or punish her, but to love her. This act, of reconnecting with the child I once was, served to validate us both, not only bridging the gaps between present and past, but also healing the fractures between them.

Through shadow work, I dance with the different parts of myself, slipping into the multitude of selves, each with its own revelation: the suppressed dreamer, the silenced truth-teller, the neglected nurturer—all facets of myself that deserved recognition. Each exploration a tribute to the fluidity and expansiveness of being. The many versions that manifest are dynamic, but in their truth they are consistent. I find strength in this openness, the capacity to inhabit various roles, to sample different energies without becoming defined by them.

The work is subtle, often quiet, like the shift of light across a room that indicates the day is nearing its end. It is not the kind of work that announces itself, but rather the kind that unfolds, layer by layer, in the silent conversations that I have with myself. It requires a certain surrender, a willingness to explore the spaces within that may not be free from suffering but are rich with story that feels like a remembered language.

15

UNFINISHED BUSINESS

Therefore, dark past,
I'm about to do it.
I'm about to forgive you
for everything.

—Mary Oliver

December 3, 2019

Mom, it's been twenty years since our last exchange,
a lifetime of silence that holds the echoes of a little
girl's voice. I haven't written to you since I was young,
maybe eleven or twelve. As I pick up my pen now,
the intention behind these words differs greatly from
the innocence of my earlier letters. I'm no longer
desperate for you to be well. Or to really see me and
be inspired to change. I'm not writing to beg you to
let me help you (as if I could). Or to stop hurting

me. I'm not even asking you to acknowledge that you have a problem or that you weren't there for all of those years. I won't be sliding this letter under your bedroom door, hoping you'll read it and respond, even in anger.

Aside from my face and maybe my voice, I imagine I'd be unrecognizable to you. My life looks so different from anything you know. I have been morphed through decades of seeking and seeing, of learning the sacred act of mothering myself that eluded me for many years. Since our paths diverged, my journey has been a montage of challenges and blessings, a patchwork quilt of hardship and healing. Today, I find myself in the embrace of solitude—no longer haunted by self-loathing, free from the inner voices that once posed as my own. Gone are the days of filling my hours with distractions to shield myself from emotions I feared might consume me. I stand unburdened, confronting pain without flinching. There's only me now.

I've nearly reached the age you were when our paths diverged. A lifetime has passed in these past twenty years. The ceaseless ache of losing you, the cycle of obsession over not having you, the haunting question of whether I ever truly did—I'm releasing it all. I am profoundly grateful for the person this loss has forged within me, but my life can't revolve around it anymore. I can no longer tether my existence to the idea of you, to be cruel to myself or to hide from the world. Loneliness, abandonment, the weight of this abstract connection—I relinquish them too. I have grown strong for having carried such heavy feelings for as long as I did, but I also have felt so much pain, a hunger for which there can be no satiable offering. To not know your present, nurturing, unconditional love. To only know neglect and feel an absence greater than your presence. To wrestle with the legacy of being left behind. And to know that I can be whole even with the hole you left in me. I can nurture the love within me that you couldn't provide. And it's okay. I am okay.

I've learned that contentment and joy can co-exist with the pain that has shaped me. I have made space for the glorious and the excruciating to dance together. And in the serenity of my solitude, I have learned to love the woman I chose to become. It is time for me to embrace her fully, to stand completely in the sun, unencumbered by the long shadow of your absence. And to do that, I have to let you go. Please, let me go too.

With love and liberation,
Daria

I had a vivid, recurring dream that placed my mother and me together in the familiar yet distorted setting of my old neighborhood. The streets are shrouded in twilight, that in-between light that neither promises the hope of day nor the surrender of night. We are walking side by side, but she remains half a step ahead, just slightly out of reach. Her face is clear and unlined, a picture of the past frozen in time, while mine reflects the years of living she's missed. We talk about mundane things, nothing I ever recall. Her voice is always distant. She seems absorbed by something out of sight. "I'll be right back," she says, and disappears. Moments pass and she reemerges. As I approach her, I see that her attention is fixed on something she's trying to hide. But she's not able to conceal from me that she is holding a small bag of crack.

In another dream we are driving together, and she asks to make a "quick stop." She leaves me to wait in the car as she goes into a building. The waiting grows tiresome, and I decide to go in and get her. I enter and navigate a series of rooms that all look exactly alike. Eventually, I find her, and she's huddled with a group of people, usually men I don't recognize, and they're doing drugs. I call out to her, trying to bridge the few physical steps between us that feel like miles, but she doesn't hear me. When she realizes I'm there, she reacts like a child who has just been caught eating dessert before dinner and insists that she "isn't doing anything." In every version of the dream, I am always reaching out, trying to grasp her, to save her, but my hands close on air.

Waking from these dreams, the morning light offers no relief. Instead, I'm disoriented by a lingering sadness that covers me like a blanket. This sadness gradually evaporates to reveal anger—not just with her for her repeated failures, but with myself for my subconscious longing that things could have been different. This hope, which never saw the light of day, seems futile and foolish.

For years, I'd had these dreams and was aware of the unresolved feelings toward my mother that were surfacing in my subconscious. But I had felt unequipped to approach them until the day in 2019 when I dug up my three-year-old copy of *Mothers Who Can't Love: A Healing Guide for Daughters* by Susan Forward, PhD, best-selling author and therapist, who worked with hundreds of women who grew up with abusive mothers. After having one such dream, I bought Forward's book with the goal of understanding and making peace with my mother's behavior. However, it sat on the shelf unread, and then in a moving box that would travel with me from Providence back to New York and then to LA, after I left Facebook for a role as chief marketing officer at JustFab.

A few months prior, I'd gone back to Detroit for the graduation of my youngest niece, Taylor, at the Detroit Opera House, where my own graduation had been held. In the twilight zone between familial duty and personal autonomy, I began staying at hotels when visiting, a decision necessitated by my sister's expanding household after the arrival of her fourth child in 2008.

I hadn't bothered to confirm the guest list, assuming it mirrored the one from Rory's graduation two years prior: Leah, Samuel (my sister's ex-husband), the three non-graduating kids, their paternal grandmother, and perhaps some random friends of my sister—that was the expected lineup.

I sat on the aisle next to Rory, and Leah sat next to her. Samuel was behind us with my nephews. My father, known for his belated appearances, joined late, securing a seat somewhere in the periphery. But my mother, slipping in just before the ceremony, settled some twenty seats away at the opposite end of our row. It's uncertain whether she saw me, as she left before the ceremony concluded, right after Taylor crossed the stage.

A familiar pang, reminiscent of a past departure at my own graduation, resurfaced. My stomach began to turn, and I feared Taylor would exit the auditorium looking for her, as I had in 1998, when she left in the middle of my high school graduation. Those of us in my dance company who were graduating performed as part of the ceremony, our very last together, so I had to be at the theater early. This would be the first time my mother had ever seen me perform. Our dance company had done recitals all over the city and even at an international dance festival in Miami, but my mother had never seen me onstage. We performed a lyrical piece to Deniece Williams's "Black Butterfly" before joining our classmates in the auditorium for the speeches. After the ceremony, we made our way to the atrium and hugged one another while searching for our respective families. I spotted Leah, who was standing alone, and made my way to her.

"Heeey!" I said cheerfully, while scanning the area for Mom.

"Hey. Mama left," Leah said with just a hint of incredulity.

On the verge of tears, I choked up a response. "She left? When? Where did she go?"

"I don't know. A while ago. She just left and told me to get a ride home with you and Marcus."

Marcus was my high school boyfriend. We became friends the first semester of our junior year and started dating winter term. He and his family had moved from Dallas for his father's job, so he transferred to my high school. Renaissance required an entrance exam and application and was the most competitive of the three schools of its kind, but his father, Dr. Curtis Ivery, had been the youngest and the first Black person appointed to serve in the cabinet of then governor Bill Clinton, and in 1996, was recruited to Detroit as the chancellor of the Wayne County Community College District. Marcus also had his own car—a two-year-old Jeep Grand Cherokee that his mother drove before Dr. Ivery bought her a new Mercedes E-Class—and was always picking me up or dropping me off at home, even though he lived all the way downtown and our apartment building was about ten minutes past school in the other direction. But we were already downtown, making it a significant detour to take us home when he practically lived down the street.

"What? He is going out with his family to celebrate. I don't know if he can take us all the way to Southfield and make it back here in time."

It took me a while to find Marcus, despite his six-foot-four-inch height. As I looked for him, I encountered other friends and classmates, congratulating them and introducing Leah, who went to a different high school. I held back tears when anyone asked where my parents were or if we were going out to eat after. Graduation party invitations had already been extended, so no one asked if I was having one. No one knew about my tumultuous home situation, and I was intent on keeping them in the dark. I think I lied and said my mother was sick and had to leave early. I don't remember giving any excuse for my father. I eventually saw Marcus and made my way to him, explaining that my mother had left and asking if he could drive us home. He was happy to do so; he had the time, and he knew I'd be stranded otherwise. That familiar ache of abandonment crept in, tainting the moment I had envisioned as a triumph for both me and my family.

In her book, Forward introduces "the five common varieties of mothers who can't love"—the Severely Narcissistic Mother, the Overly Enmeshed Mother, the Control Freak Mother, the Mother Who Needs Mothering, and the

Mother Who Neglects, Betrays, and Batters. Through stories from therapy sessions with her former patients, she illustrates the resulting mother wounds that each type tends to inflict. It was an affirming and at times painful read, as I saw my mother in several categories. I stopped reading many times before I could finish.

One of the most powerful tools I discovered in the book was a letter-writing exercise. Forward advises writing a letter that follows a four-part structure: (1) this is what you did to me, (2) this is how I felt about it at the time, (3) this is how it affected my life, and (4) this is what I want from you now. Then she recommends sharing it with a trusted person. I wrote my letter just after my thirty-ninth birthday, but I wasn't ready to share it with anyone until now.

It was also around this time that I began private Pilates reformer sessions with a trainer. My first exposure to the practice had been in high school, where our dance warm-ups and recovery sessions were based on mat Pilates. But I hadn't spent much time on the reformer, and it had been a while. Age and years of comfort bingeing along with wining and dining clients had started to show. When I first began working with Dara, I was self-conscious, acutely aware of every extra pound, every spot where my body had swelled and softened.

I walked into the group fitness studio in my apartment building, greeted by four reformers waiting for me. The space was bright and airy with two-story ceilings, bathed in natural light streaming through the exterior door and large windows. It was quintessentially LA. I arrived before Dara, so I pulled two reformers out from the corner and set them up in the middle of the room. We had been working together three times a week for the past six weeks and I knew the drill.

"Good morning! How are you?" Dara asked as I took my sneakers off.

"Still waking up," I replied with a sarcastic smile. It had been dark out when my alarm went off and the sun was still rising. I didn't love 6 a.m. sessions, but I loved having them done before the workday started.

We started with gentle stretches. Dara guided me to focus on my breath and to knit my ribs together to keep my lower back flat on the carriage. Her voice was calm and steady, leading me through the warm-up. As we moved on to more challenging exercises, I could feel my muscles waking up and the familiar burn setting in. I pushed through, relying on the endorphins to keep me going.

We finally reached the last set of exercises. Every part of my body screamed in protest, but I stayed focused on the present moment. On the burn in my muscles, the sweat on my skin, the steady rhythm of my breath. It was another kind of meditation, a way of anchoring myself in the present. I was learning a new definition of strength. One that had less to do with endurance and more to do with intention. Less about gritting my teeth and more about learning to trust myself.

Before that session, I had been afraid to do an inversion going from a downward dog position where your hands are on the shoulder pads and your feet are on the bar into a plank. For weeks, I would put my arms on the shoulder pads and as I'd go to put my foot on the bar, I'd stop. "I can't do it. I'm going to fall." I didn't think I had the arm strength to hold myself up in the starting position, let alone to push the carriage out to plank and then repeat it. So, when Dara asked me if I was up for trying, I surprised myself when I said yes. I took my position, hands firmly planted. I placed my left foot on the bar, then the right. I shifted a bit to make sure I was steady and then I pushed and pulled back in. Six times, each one feeling easier while demanding more from me.

"You did it! How did it feel?" Dara's smile was wide.

"Kind of amazing! Strong," I said, exhilarated. "I have literally jumped out of a plane before, but I was terrified of falling on my face with that move. But now that I've done it, I feel kind of silly that I was so scared."

As we dismounted the reformers to cool down, Dara smiled. "Great session today; you looked like a pro."

I returned her smile, feeling a fleeting sense of pride. "Thank you," I said. But then, without really thinking, I added, "I definitely felt like I struggled through it. I just don't understand why this is so hard."

The words surprised me, tears welling up and spilling over.

"I don't know where that came from just now," I gasped.

Her concern was immediate, but gentle.

"What's hard?" she asked.

"All of it. I had a SoulCycle instructor who used to say, 'The push is what changes you.' I feel like I'm pushing against a wall. I'm doing everything right, and it's still so hard." I had been clinging tightly to a version of myself that no longer existed—the one who could skip meals for a week and drop five pounds, who could work out consistently and see immediate results, who treated her body like something she needed to control—when what I needed was to let go. Of my devotion to it being "too hard" to lose weight. To the story that I didn't have the same metabolism I did at twenty-five. Or thirty. To the frustration that this person can eat "whatever they want" but I can't. To the idea that not eating certain foods was deprivation rather than an act of self-care, particularly when I felt miserable after eating them. To the fierce attachments to things being harder than they need to be. To being seen through any filter other than my own.

We moved between gentle stretches. My heart rate slowed, my mind wandered. I had been going through the motions, performing someone else's prescription for wellness. Treating my body like a battlefield, enemy territory versus the ally it is. "I have to meet my body where it is today," I finally said. "Figure out what this version of me needs. It's like being reintroduced to myself."

In that moment, I became clear and intentional about what I really needed to shed. In the process, I would go on to lose forty pounds, but the real shedding had been of the mindset that kept me wanting things to be different. My mindfulness extended to my eating, an area of my life that had run on autopilot for years, dictated by the inner child who was taught to eat everything on her plate and on a schedule, rather than listening to her own body. Instead, I learned to let my hunger be the signal that it was time to eat and let the craving for comfort be the signal that I needed a walk, a hug from a friend, a call with my niece, gentler words for myself, a deeper connection with my own soul.

In navigating this new landscape of self-awareness, I felt a growing resolve to understand this wound in the shape of my mother. This meant undertaking a courageous and tender exploration of the state my mother was in when I was born, prompting me to answer a series of questions (whose origin I no longer recall) that might contextualize the wounds I had ·begun to uncover.

"What was your mother's mental state when she was pregnant with you? When you were born?"

Seriously? I had no idea. I understood the reasoning behind this question, but my inability to answer it didn't inspire confidence as I began the exercise. A silence echoed in my mind, a void where answers should have been. I had no photographs of my mother from this period, no letters she had written or fragments of her life to sift through. With a photo, I could at least have studied her eyes, searching for traces of emotion that might indicate her state of mind. She was only twenty-one when I was born. Was she anxious, excited, or perhaps a bit of both as she carried the promise of my arrival in her heart? I moved on.

"Do you know the details of your birth story?"

Jesus. I didn't know that either, only the name of the hospital where I was born and the time I arrived. I don't know if my father was there, if he drove my mother to the hospital or if Grandma had taken her. Did her water break in the middle of the grocery store or was she home when she went into labor? New questions multiplied like ripples in a pond. Did my mother hold me immediately after, feeling the weight of my tiny frame against her chest? Had there been a connection forged in those precious moments that laid the foundation for the years to come? Who cut the umbilical cord? I only knew that I had been born with a hernia, one that healed itself after a few months. The answer was always in my stomach.

"Did your mother experience postpartum depression?"

The words reverberated like an unanswered call—another unknown in a growing list. Many women endured postpartum depression in silence, I reminded myself. If the answer was yes, it is likely I would never have known, even if my mother had remained a part of my life. Yet, the question stirred deeper reflections about her life before me, particularly the loss of her own father less than a decade before my birth, and the impact it undoubtedly had on her, shaping my earliest experiences.

The research on intergenerational trauma, while still

emerging, supports the theory that traumatic experiences can cascade down through generations, not just through shared stories and mimicked behaviors, but also through biological imprints. This is the language of epigenetics, in which our personal histories are subtly inscribed into our DNA, not altering the structure of our genes, but rather influencing their expression. This profound yet understated dialogue between generations might mold everything from our vulnerability to stress to the ways in which we navigate our emotions.

As a fetus develops, it is not merely nurtured by the nutrients and oxygen delivered through the placenta; it is also subtly shaped by the mother's emotional and physiological states. If the mother experiences stress or depression, the biochemical signals of these states also travel through the umbilical cord, imprinting her emotional landscape onto the child. It is as if the daughter inherits a book from her mother, annotated not in ink but in cortisol and adrenaline, the underlined passages and folded pages marking significant emotional events that belong to the mother. Even before birth, a child's nervous system is being tuned, primed by her mother's experiences, laying a foundation that will influence her way of interacting with the world.

The implications of this are vast and nuanced, and while I grappled with these questions, I was left to consider the unspoken legacies that linger in the gaps of my own family's narrative. How much of my mother's unarticulated sorrows, her unresolved grief over her father's death, had I inherited?

These were not merely rhetorical questions but potentially, keys to understanding the layers of who I was—formed by the unseen forces of a past that was not solely my own.

Did your parents have a healthy relationship?

I knew they hadn't, but I didn't know when their problems began or the extent. They were married for three years before I was born. They had moved to Ohio or maybe Kentucky while my father was still in the army, but my mother returned to Detroit shortly after she discovered she was pregnant. I think she went back alone. The specifics of their life together—the places they shared before the duplex on Ohio Street, whether they even lived there together or if we moved there after they broke up, the exact moment my father might have drifted from the picture—were all unknowns.

I set the pen down in my open journal in an admission of defeat. The questions stared back at me, demanding a clarity I could not provide. I had failed a test about my own life.

More than the scarcity of facts, what had become clear to me was the abundance of absence, the profound presence of what was not there. This emptiness had surely shaped me as profoundly as the physical DNA that coursed through my veins. It was a different kind of genetic code, one written in the fears and feelings I'd worked to overcome.

The not knowing gnawed at me, but I allowed time to pass, hoping that with distance, more details might emerge. Days turned to weeks, before I found myself drawn back to the task. In the optimism of a new attempt, I faced the questions again. Nothing. I retreated again from the pursuit, my mother's absence a silent presence in every answer I struggled to give.

There were times I pitied my mother, recognizing the magnitude of her suffering. But as an adult, I have chosen not to be a witness to her journey, to watch her struggle to piece herself together. No one wants to see their mother suffer, and I spent too many years mothering her. The instinct to take a leading role would be too great. Mostly, I resented her—her weaknesses, her squandered potential. I redirected my feelings about her into quiet anger, suppressing and repressing them, and ultimately, projecting them onto her and anyone who reminded me of her. I blamed her for being the source of my pain and the architect of her own ruin and judged her for her inability to admit it.

But compassion, when it came, arrived not as a sudden epiphany but as a byproduct of the grace I began to extend to myself. Pema Chödrön teaches that "compassion is not a relationship between the healer and the wounded. It's a relationship between equals. Only when we know our own darkness well can we be present with the darkness of others." I don't know if I would call it forgiveness or even true understanding. Both terms feel simultaneously loaded and reductive. For years, I wrestled with how and whether to forgive my parents for failing to be the caregivers I needed. I had always heard that forgiveness is the only way to free yourself. *Forgive unless you want to be imprisoned in your own pain.*

To do otherwise is like drinking poison and waiting for the other person to die. But emotionally, this is a Herculean task. Promising forgiveness feels like a setup. Our socialization all but demands that reconciliation be the highest form of forgiveness. Reconciling with my parents would first mean that they needed to do the work to get sober and to heal. I could never count on this.

What happens next looks something like this: You grieve the loss of the parents you never had, lamenting the absence of a functional family, the advice that was never imparted, the comforting embraces that were too rare, and the supportive words that were never spoken. It's a grieving for what could have been while contending with the emotions that arise as you listen to people talk about family, thinking how much they take for granted—that they'll see each other again soon, that they'd have holidays together, that the other would be just a phone call away. To know the feeling of going "home" to people who know you as well as you know yourself. It will never cease to amaze me how people speak of family as an ordinary blessing. I guess it's easy to decide that family is common when you have it.

Next, you mourn your parents' inability to experience the lives they must have once dreamed of. My mother never made use of the gifts she was born with. She graduated from high school when she was fifteen, but because Grandma didn't think she was ready for college, her education was put on hold, and she got modeling jobs in local runway shows and print ads for some of Detroit's small businesses. At some point, she enrolled in a nursing program, but it seems that aspiration may have gotten lost somewhere in the married at eighteen and two kids by twenty-two of it all. I have allowed myself to briefly imagine how her life might have unfolded had she gone to school. In this alternate universe, her dreams are not casualties of circumstance; they are the engines of her triumph. And as her child, I grow up not under the shadow of her limitations, but in the light of her achievements, my own path illuminated by the example of her brilliance. I don't entertain it for long, but I grieve for the woman she would never become. I mourn for the art she never created, the dreams she never chased, and the tranquility she never found. For the loss of what could have enriched the world, and for my never getting to witness it.

I'm left with the pauses and silences of my parents' lives, their losses and joys never fully seen but forever felt. Perhaps their unrealized potential includes the parents they wish they could have been. My mother raised me from her wounds, not her scars. Maybe that was honest effort.

Ultimately, though, it was my responsibility to deal with my *own* feelings more than to make sense of hers. It's a strange thing to recognize, but I can't blame my parents for their weaknesses any more than I can blame myself for the consequences of those weaknesses. (Having terrible parents isn't a prerequisite for developing misconceptions and defensive strategies, by the way.)

More than anything, you grieve for the inner child who lives inside of you.

And it all amounts to something that looks like acceptance—not as resignation but as an embrace. This acceptance does not demand resolution or reconciliation but an acknowledgment that empty spaces may remain.

༄

"For months, I have been wrestling with this inner child exercise," I explained to Erin, the therapist I began seeing after moving to LA. "It starts with these questions about my mother's pregnancy, my birth, whether she suffered postpartum depression, and I can't answer any of them."

She listened, her eyes reflecting the complexity of my exploration. "What do you feel like you would accomplish if you were to complete it?"

"Well, it's part of my inner child healing work. I thought if I could understand the emotional state my mother was in when I was born, and other details about my early life, it might help me uncover any subconscious beliefs I have." I had chosen to work with Erin in part because she specialized in trauma and EMDR therapy and utilized a number of the modalities that I had employed on my own, including visualization, breathwork, and mindfulness exercises.

"Would having the answers about her emotional state change your ability to do that work?" she gently pushed.

"No," I conceded. There was no case to be made.

"Can you be okay if you never get the answers?" Erin asked, guiding me to the heart of my struggle.

I sat with it for a moment and a quiet acceptance emerged—a realization that I could locate a different kind of peace, a way to be whole despite the missing pieces of my beginnings.

"I have to be."

I persisted in forming an identity in light of this absence, creating an image for myself to fill in the gaps. For many years, I defined myself in opposition to my parents: I was successful despite being the daughter of addicts, and success had been my rebellion against them. I thought every straight-A report card and geometry trophy brought me one step closer to my freedom. The trouble was, I was still defining myself based on who they were, with my wounded parts at the center of this identity. Their parental neglect and the drive it spurred in me. My parents, especially my mother, were right there, at the core of who I thought I was choosing to be. For my entire childhood, my focus had been on her, becoming an expert in her needs rather than my own. I spent so much time trying to make sense of what had happened to me. It was time to once again imagine who else I might become. The ties had been cut, not cleanly with a knife, but roughly, like tearing bread with your bare hands.

I suspect there will always be a small part of me that aches to be cared for by my parents. That feeling may never go away. I'm no longer asking it to. Reparenting my inner child meant creating a functional family within myself, building a home in my heart where every part of me is welcomed, cared for, loved. It means setting a table where my inner child is always the guest of honor, where her need for beauty is celebrated, where our cravings for solo dance parties and slow mornings, walking through cities and being near the beach, are priorities. Where my needs for lengthy journaling sessions, indie French films, effortless exercise, and in-depth conversations are indulged. Much of my healing has come in hours spent doing yard work, or on my favorite hiking trails.

The last dream I had of my mother was different from the rest. We were on our way to some vague destination together, and she asked me to detour and take her somewhere else. But this time, nothing happened. There was no plummet in my stomach, no disappearance, no betrayal. I woke not in sorrow or anger, but with a sense of neutrality.

That morning, stepping into the shower, I let the water cleanse me, washing away the old narratives that had once haunted me. As I emerged and stood in front of the bathroom mirror, I considered my reflection—the few freckles that line my mother's apple cheekbones and dot my father's button nose, my own square jaw and full eyebrows, dark, and slightly feral—and I noticed a softness. Or perhaps a quiet authority that was newfound. It was not a return to what was lost, but a brave step into what might be.

16

GREY MATTER

I went from having nightmares about my mother to seeing my dead grandmother's name in an array of peculiar places. Like secret messages from beyond, her name appeared for months on boxes of biscuits at Whole Foods, on a street sign in Silver Lake, in the name of a stationery brand and the style names of a sofa and a designer tweed jacket, and then, in the name of a trade organization that invited me to be a judge for their annual marketing awards. This series of sightings wouldn't have merited attention if it were a common name like Elizabeth or Shirley or Rose. But Effie was of a rare vintage, a relic of a bygone era that defied such ordinary occurrences. Her name had always been a curiosity to me, especially in light of her younger siblings' alliterative and far more common names, Cliff and Claudia. The question of how her parents came upon Effie would remain unanswerable, another riddle from the past occupying my thoughts once again.

As the sightings multiplied, I found myself in a state of amusement and unease. Each one solicited a response that revealed itself in the strained corners of my mouth and the hesitant glimmer in my eyes. Her visitations, like seeds, had their own season to sprout, pushing through when least expected, calling for daylight and air. She had returned from the past—in name and in spirit—hovering in my present, cementing her presence into every corner of my life.

After Grandma died, my mother said she began seeing signs that she was still with us—lights flickering off and on, the blades of a still ceiling fan moving only in the shadow on the ceiling. It was one of the few things that seemed to make sense to her, to offer her solace in the depths of her grief. Even though I was just past my seventh birthday, these ghost stories didn't scare me, nor did I fear that my mother had lost her mind. I was jealous. I didn't see Grandma. She didn't come to me in my dreams or flicker the lights for me.

For years, I clung to the intangible threads that connected us. In that fragile space where the living yearn to stay with their departed. Freshman year of college was the first time I saw the cardinal, outside my dorm room window, and I decided it was a sign—an omen that she was somehow near. I had just come back from class when I saw the crimson flash in my periphery. It was early autumn, when the leaves turned from green to gold to rust, and then proceeded to cover the lawns across Ann Arbor. There it was, perched on one of the many great oak trees outside of my fifth-floor window in the back of Mary Markley Hall. We called them redbirds as little kids, marveling at the winged flames and the audacious crest on their head. I remember learning their formal name in third grade, the year I learned to spell *encyclopedia.* I learned that only males bore the vibrant signature red color that is most often associated with cardinals. This time, I looked up the spiritual significance of the northern cardinal. I did not find much back then, but what I did see consistently said that in cultures throughout history, the red cardinal is embraced as a spiritual messenger sent by our loved ones to say that they will always feel our love and will always be with us. It was a comforting thought, but not one I gave much energy to.

Over the years, the red-winged emissary followed me from Ann Arbor to Houston to Washington, DC, to New York City, and eventually, to East Hampton and Los Angeles, flashing outside the windows of each new home. "Hi, Grandma," I'd say, convinced it was her, even though I had not yet decided whether or not I even believed in reincarnation.

Effie name sightings, however, were a different matter. Surely these were not "bereavement hallucinations," the sensory perceptions like hugs or taps on the shoulder people have reported feeling after the death of a loved one. But they felt like pings from the universe that I could neither dismiss nor decipher. I began to wonder if these love taps were Grandma trying to send me another message, awaken me to something more. I documented each sighting in my journal, detailing the date, time, and location, hoping to see a pattern I might decode. And for a brief moment, I had allowed myself to believe that perhaps the internet might have the answer: "What does it mean to keep seeing a dead person's name?" I asked Google.

In the midst of this peculiar mystery, I tethered myself to the tangible world and the dreams I still had the power to shape. My mind settled into a calmer, more present state, and my body lighter from shedding the weight of old feelings, my soul craved something more.

I had always envisioned something serene and full of promise beneath my front windows at the beach house— a congregation of big white hydrangea bushes, their round heads heavy with bloom against the muted tones of my gray cedar shingle home. That spring, I texted Jamie, the landscaper who had spent the past two years helping me transform my front and side entrances with privet and boxwoods and herringbone-patterned walkways. I asked if he could stop by to discuss my next project.

"I think it's time for the hydrangeas," I explained, feeling a thrill at voicing the thought aloud. "You know it's been my dream to plant them here under the front windows. What do you think?"

"Ah, Miss Daria," he said, using the name that somehow made me feel both independent and cared for, "yes, they will be beautiful there. When do you want to start?"

"In the next month or so?" My heart swelled with anticipation.

"Okay. You got it, Miss Daria," Jamie assured me. "What kind do you want?"

"Blushing Brides," I began, my tone mirroring the certainty of my choice, "with the full round heads, or other white ones if you can't find those. Limelight, maybe?"

"I will try, Miss Daria. The soil's pH is what makes the color. If it's too acidic, they turn blue. For white, we need the soil to be just right."

I crossed my arms, a furrow creasing my brow. "So you're saying the environment dictates their color?" I mused aloud, finding the deeply resonant metaphor within his horticultural lesson.

"Yes, exactly," he confirmed. "But don't worry, I have some ways to keep the soil how we need it."

I smiled at the thought of being able to nudge them toward the destiny we envisioned for them.

"We'll give them what they need to do well." Jamie's assurance felt like a gentle pat on the back from the universe.

"Thank you, Jamie. I trust you to plant them while I'm in LA. I can't wait to see them!" My heart hitched at the idea of not being there to witness the transformation, but the trust I had in Jamie was as solid as the oaks that lined the yard.

As I headed back east a few months later, I imagined that their white blooms had by now started to unfurl. But as the house came into view, my heart lurched. Where there should have been burgeoning bushes cradling orbs of snow-white blossoms, there was only chaos. The hydrangeas had been ravaged by deer, their stems jagged and bare, leaves chewed to lace. I had envisioned a fortress of beauty; instead, I found only the ruins of a dream.

"Jamie." I sighed his name like a betrayal, feeling the sting of trust misplaced. He had assured me all would be well. Yet here stood the evidence, stark against the sun-bleached wood—nature had defied us both. I texted him and asked if he could come by the next day.

"Oh my God. Wow." Jamie's voice, usually more robust, now carried an edge of trepidation. "I sprayed for deer every week. It must have just happened. I—I didn't think they would come. Not this close to the house."

"Neither did I," I said, my voice now absent of accusation yet full of disappointment. "I am so sad, Jamie. Are they gone forever? Can they come back?"

After a moment, he said, "Yes, they can grow back, but not here."

I stood there, the question of what to do next resting heavy on my shoulders like a sodden wool blanket. I didn't want to waste any more time or money until I had a plan. I asked Jamie to cover them in the meantime. I knew this was but a temporary solution—a bandage on a deeper wound. Jamie wrapped the bushes in burlap with meticulous care, shrouding them from further destruction. It was an act of protection, a gesture of hope against the elements and invaders.

As I watched him work, I couldn't help but think about the lengths we go to cultivate the new and the measures we take to protect what we cherish. Whether wrapping fragile beginnings in burlap or preserving the delicate parts of ourselves, each act shows our deep desire to hold on to what we love, even as the world seems intent on taking it away.

Standing there, watching the hydrangeas being carefully covered, I felt a stirring within me, an undeniable urge to protect and nurture my own spirit. The hydrangeas were not just plants; they were symbols of the life I yearned to cultivate, a life that required stepping away from the familiar confines of the chief marketing officer role that had taken me to Los Angeles two years prior. After twenty years in marketing and reaching fashion's C-suite, I was suddenly clear that it was time for a change. I had said an unwavering "yes" to what I thought was a dream job, and in some ways, it was. But I was no longer guided by a dysregulated nervous system that said I needed to prove myself by pushing as hard as I could. I was being pulled by the potential of something else, something more. The path I had been following disappeared and I was on my way.

I decided to resign from my role and take my first fearless bold step into the unknown. I rented an apartment in the eighth arrondissement, steps away from the famous Rue du Faubourg Saint-Honoré. This was an unprecedented move for me, someone who seldom took more than a week's vacation. But I intuitively knew Paris was where I needed to be. I have long considered Paris a "soul home" that feels as essential to me as New York. I had visited several times before, but always in brief, tantalizing glances. The idea of an extended stay had been a recurring fantasy, thwarted during business school by practicalities and the fear of missing out on life back home—Jake, my friends, opportunities that seemed too precious to leave behind. Now was my chance to heed the call of what my soul was asking me to do.

I didn't plan a set itinerary ahead of time. Instead, my goal was to embrace slow living, to wake up each morning and ask, "What does my soul need today?" I was being called to turn my ear inward and to hear the answers to this question without the noise of deliverables, deadlines, or productivity. Maybe I'd hear Grandma too. For the first time in my life, I would avail myself fully to whatever came to me in silent conversations with my own heart.

I felt in myself a yearning to open a door through which something just beyond my grasp might live, so before my departure, I made another meaningful decision—to get a SPECT (single photon emission computed tomography) scan at the renowned Amen Clinics in Los Angeles, founded by Dr. Daniel Amen, a psychiatrist and brain researcher on a mission to push the boundaries of neurophysiology and advance the landscape of brain health. My first encounter with Dr. Amen's work had occurred a couple of years earlier, so the thought had had plenty of time to marinate.

I lay on the padded table, eyes fixed on the top of the

scanner, questions racing through my mind. I attempted to concentrate on my breath while a gamma camera captured 120 detailed images of my brain, spanning a 360-degree rotation in three-degree increments. The rhythmic tapping of the scanner filled the room, a metronome marking time as I waited for it to end. Uncertainty clung to me. *I don't know what I don't know.* But I reminded myself that the body holds the answers to our most deeply held questions. I had collected four years of evidence by then. Closing my eyes again, I slipped into the dark room of my mind. My thoughts incessantly strayed to this idea: *What if, hidden in my biology, lurks something I don't know about? What of my childhood has been imprinted on me?* This felt like the final step in my research, out of my books and under the skin.

At forty, I had long ago dismissed the possibility of addiction manifesting in my own being. The first time I took a shot, at a bar with colleagues from my first job out of college, I stood there waiting to turn into the Incredible Hulk (or my mother). I was twenty, and my only experience with drinking before that involved two glasses of wine at a special dinner to celebrate my college boyfriend's law firm job offer. Nothing much happened either time, aside from feeling a bit giddy. The first time I got hammered was a night a couple of years later when I was twenty-three. Hoping to cultivate a "sophisticated" cocktail palate, I had one too many pomegranate margaritas over dinner with a friend at Rosa Mexicano in Washington, DC. The swift taxi ride home led to me sitting on the cold bathroom floor cradling the toilet bowl with both arms while the room spun, praying to God that I hadn't become an alcoholic. I traced the lines of my hands, wondering if the same demons that haunted my parents lurked inside of me and whether I could look them in the face and survive if they surfaced.

If I were destined to become an addict, surely it would have happened before I turned forty, right? *Right?* I latched on to this thought with the determination of a hungry newborn. Still, the thoughts came: *What if the demons that haunted my parents and both of my grandfathers dwell within me? How many generations of alcohol-soaked, drug-dependent chromosomes lay dormant, poised to surface without warning?* "Alcohol and drug addiction doesn't come in bottles. It doesn't even come in your DNA. It comes in people." I remembered reading that somewhere.

With a roster of high-profile patients, Dr. Amen himself has become a bit of a celebrity. His unconventional approach of peering into the brain itself when considering a patient's mental and behavioral health struck me as both innovative and compelling. His belief—like that of Doidge, van der Kolk, Dr. Leah Swart, and the many neuroscientists and psychiatrists I had studied—that "you can literally change people's brains," and his dedication, demonstrated through the scrutiny of more than one hundred thousand SPECT scans, held the promise of insight and transformation.

Amen's Encino-based clinic stood in stark contrast to

what I had come to expect from a "celebrity" doctor's office. In a far cry from many of the sleek offices I had seen in New York City and Beverly Hills, the receptionist was seated behind plexiglass, enclosed in what looked like a small conference room. Warm beige walls and fluorescent lighting intensified the dissonance. Muted gray chairs bore wooden arms that matched the floor-to-ceiling bookcases that held Dr. Amen's books and supplements, an altar to his life's work.

After signing in for my appointment, I had been greeted by a technician who escorted me to a quiet, dimly lit room. There, I sat in silence for fifteen minutes after she injected a small amount of radioactive tracer into my bloodstream. The tracer, designed to highlight areas of heightened brain activity, called for two brain scans. The first, a resting scan to establish a baseline for my brain activity; the second, to observe the brain in action. For the resting scan, I was instructed to do nothing. I was prohibited from closing my eyes, falling asleep, even meditating. I sat, trying to think of nothing. Then trying not to try. Every action, no matter how insignificant, seemed to constitute as brain activity. Determined not to contaminate my results, I managed to zone out. The technician came back and escorted me to another room where she would scan my brain. This time, I lay on the X-ray table, assuming the position of a patient on a medical TV show. Allowing my body's full weight to rest on the table, I lay impossibly still while the camera captured images of my brain.

The next day, the same technician escorted me to the same dark room, again injecting the tracer—this time before leaving me to take a fourteen-minute concentration study. I sat for the Conners Continuous Performance Test (CCPT), my eyes fixated on a computer screen, where I was instructed to respond whenever any letter appeared—except for the letter X. By evaluating performance in areas of inattentiveness, impulsivity, sustained attention, and vigilance, psychiatrists use the CCPT to aid in the diagnosis of attention deficit hyperactivity disorder (ADHD) and other psychological and neurological conditions related to attention.

The process culminated in a two-hour brain assessment, a standardized series of tests to evaluate risk of mental health conditions along with performance across the dimensions of emotion, feeling, cognition, and self-control.

I would have to wait months for the results. It was August, and the doctor I would be working with wasn't available to meet with me until late November. While waiting for the results, I decided to leave LA for a few months to enjoy a change of scenery. On Labor Day, I flew to New York and spent the rest of the month in East Hampton. Friends drove or took the train out for weekend visits, and I caught up with others in the city. Three weeks evaporated, a blur of familiar faces and conversations that danced around the edges of my excitement. It was all preparation for what was to come—a month and a half in Paris.

Arriving in Paris is always like stepping into a memory

half dreamed, half remembered. A place where the line between the real and the imagined dissolves. But my first few days were marked by incessant rain. I wandered the apartment, shifting from window to window, from the sofa to the chair, watching the droplets race down the glass, unable to settle on anything. By day four, I remembered my commitment to embrace slow living and spontaneity. I began each day with a ninety-minute routine of journaling, stretching, and meditating, followed by one introspective question: "What do I need today?" And I would wait until the answer came to me. Some days, the only obvious thing to do was walk.

My initiation into the church of walking had occurred when I first arrived in Ann Arbor. The University of Michigan's campus was a revelation after growing up in Detroit, where slow encounters were seldom invited. From the mix of Greek and Neo-Renaissance Revival architecture on Central Campus to the quaint charm of downtown Ann Arbor, to the tranquil paths in "the Arb," I discovered how the simple heel-to-toe gesture repeated in tandem can shake loose the stubborn thoughts that cling to the corners of our minds.

On those solitary walks, I unearthed the profound connection between mind and feet, which became a path to some kind of clarity for me, especially after my mother disappeared. For me, in moments of feeling down or stuck or lost, there's often a voice within, calling for movement, for change, for evolution. Walking is always my answer to that call. Each step sets the mind and the soul in motion, and walking becomes a portal for processing, reflection, and giving ourselves space to expand. It's as much a cognitive journey as it is a physical one, an opportunity to unpack the thoughts and experiences of the day, and sometimes, to let them go. I walk to find out what I'm thinking and what it means. Each walk in Paris was a ceremony of reconnection, a deliberate pilgrimage to a sacred space within myself. This, too, is integration.

One evening, I met up with my friend Jen, who was in Paris on business. Halfway through dinner and a bottle of pinot noir, the topic of my mother arose.

"How long has it been since you last spoke to your mother?" Jen asked.

"Almost nineteen years," I said, refilling my wineglass. The words hung there, a prophecy of the space that stretched between us. A gulf filled with milestones she wouldn't witness, heartaches I would navigate alone, and triumphs bittersweet for lack of sharing. But within that gap, I would do the work of uncovering the wounds, untethering from old stories, and meeting the needs that had long been silenced.

"I didn't realize it had been that long. That's a long time," she said, her eyes searching for my feelings about it. "And she has never reached out?"

"Once, maybe a year into our estrangement?" I took a sip. "I told her that as long as she was unwell and not willing to acknowledge it or how it's affected me, I couldn't have her in my life. And I told her not to call me again. And she just said, 'Okay.'"

"That must be hard." I heard sympathy for me and my mother. "For you to go all of those years without your mom, and for a mother to go all those years without seeing her child...to honor your wishes like that, maybe that was her showing you how much she loves you. That you expressed that as your greatest need at the time and it was something she could actually give you."

I had never once thought of it that way. That her ultimate act of love was her willingness to let me go because that was what I needed. I cleared my throat trying to catch the tears welling up before one could spill over.

17

STILL PROCESSING

As my last days in Paris approached, I was surprised to find that I felt neither desperate to leave nor to stay. It was just time to go back home. I flew to New York, where I spent a few days before heading back to LA. I kept waiting to fall back into my old routine, the way you tend to once you're home from vacation, but I never did. Something had changed.

I had gone away without an agenda, but the unstructured time had been a six-week meditation of sorts, and I returned with a deep sense of clarity having reconnected with myself. For four years I had become obsessed with making some kind of sense of my suffering and my survival. I had studied it from every angle. But this exploration had been largely theoretical, removed from the act of living. I got caught in a cycle of self-analysis, barricaded behind insights that only told part of the story.

In December, I returned to the clinic for my meeting with Dr. Brush, a naturopathic doctor at Amen Clinics whose approach to mental health considers the holistic well-being of a person. When I asked to work with Dr. Brush, it was her desire to address the mental, physical, emotional, biochemical, and spiritual aspects of a person's life and her experience with addiction treatment that resonated with me. She seemed like someone who could consider my family history in the context of my brain scans. Perhaps she held a key to unlocking not only my brain's secrets, but the echoes of generations past. In our ninety-minute session, Dr. Brush would reveal the intricacies of my brain scans and the assessments I'd taken and provide recommendations for sustaining my brain and mental health. And now, arriving at Amen Clinics again after the time that had passed, I felt little more than curiosity.

I scribbled my name on the sign-in sheet and sat briefly in the company of a father and daughter who were also waiting to be seen. The girl looked tall for her age, no more than thirteen. And I remembered that Dr. Amen was board-certified in both general and child psychiatry. *I hope she's okay,* I thought to myself, an offering of compassion for her unknown struggles, also recognizing the fortune of having a parent who cared enough to have brought her there. Medical waiting rooms have a remarkable way of eliciting empathy and gratitude for the shared human experience.

Dr. Brush greeted me with a warm welcome and led me to her office. She had a slender frame and a posture that suggested a devotion to yoga. Her black pantsuit struck me as quite formal for a naturopathic doctor who has lived and worked in Oregon, Hawaii, and California. She sat at her desk with a bookcase behind her that featured an array of psychology and neuroscience books, along with a 3D model of the brain. I refrained from asking her if I could have a closer look. *It's not a toy, Daria.* On the wall to her right hung a lovely landscape painting of the ocean, and I wondered if she had selected it or if the art choices were predetermined by whoever decorated the clinic. As she spoke, Dr. Brush reflected the wisdom of the ocean—deep, knowing, accepting—and I decided that it had been her choice.

She began our discussion by inquiring about my motivation for seeking a brain scan. I quickly recounted my journey of the past four years—the photograph of the accident, my subsequent fascination with neuroscience and psychology, neuroplasticity and epigenetics, and my pursuit to understand myself through the unique lens that only a brain scan might offer.

"My friends—at least the ones who know I'm doing this—are certainly intrigued, but they also think I'm a bit... out there sometimes," I said, careful not to say "crazy" or "insane."

Dr. Brush explained the scoring system of the first test, the CCPT.

"These might be the best set of results I've seen in the past six months! You have an excellent ability to focus and concentrate on a task. But I'm not surprised. You performed well academically, and typically, people who do so do not have a big problem with attention and focus. Let's look at your total brain assessment."

"I actually took the assessment twice."

"How did that happen?"

"Well...the always/never questions always trip me up! Like, is once in the past year *almost never*, or is it *occasionally*?" The overachiever in me wanted to get the answers right.

Dr. Brush laughed easily, but it was clear I would not get much banter back from her. "No worries. Your standardized scores look really good. No signs of substance abuse. No signs of PTSD. No signs of ADHD here either. No signs of social anxiety or sleep apnea."

The little boost to my ego was appreciated until I remembered that many of the people who went to Amen Clinics did so with concerns about their attention and cognitive function. I had not.

The next set of scores on the second report were plotted along sliding scales, the colors—green, gray, red—denoting strengths, averages, and areas of struggle. Admittedly, it was interesting to see such a complex picture of my identity, an entire narrative etched in data.

"Your scores are represented here in the bubbles." She

traced her pen over the columns and scores that mapped the landscape of my psychology, a portrait of my innermost self.

"There are three very interesting things I want to point out," she began. "First, the absence of scores in the red, which is an anomaly in itself, speaks to a certain tenacity and an ability to withstand life's challenges." Her voice carried warm undertones of knowing. I found myself wanting to channel her blend of calm authority and compassionate insight.

"Second, you have a very low negativity bias, both subconscious (ninety-fifth percentile) and conscious (ninety-first percentile). This means that adverse events have less of an effect on your psychological state than neutral or positive events. So even in the face of a challenge, you're able and likely to see the positive side of things. But look at this—" A dash of excitement seeped in, the change in her tone marking a shift in focus as she steered my attention to the next set of scores.

"You are in the ninety-eighth percentile for resilience and ninety-seventh percentile for stress control! Goodness gracious. I suspect that this is why you did not repeat the life that was modeled for you. You have an incredibly strong sense of resilience, so despite your upbringing, you were not left feeling like you had no choice. You were able to recover from multiple traumatic events and manage the stress very effectively. This, combined with your optimism and future orientation, also means that you're able to envision and move toward a positive outcome even in the face of something extremely difficult. That is rare."

"Ninety-eighth percentile for resilience and ninety-seventh

percentile for stress control?" I echoed her enthusiasm, savoring the insight. To see it quantified on paper was stunning. Official.

"This little bit of data says so much..." I said, my voice carrying the weight of reflection. "Dr. Brush, how much of this is genetic versus temperament? Or a consequence of my upbringing? I'm just thinking—would I be less resilient if the traumatic events of my life happened earlier or later? How much may have been shaped by the first seven years of life? I guess I'm asking—"

"Is it nature or nurture?" she interrupted, finishing my sentence, then flipping to the brain scans.

"Do you recall I said I can tell by looking at your brain that you likely had some childhood trauma? Well, there are two ways this shows up in your scans."

The first scan showed what Dr. Brush described as "very mild scalloping," where the brain, on the outside surface view, appears irregular and not smooth. Scalloping, she said, indicates lower blood flow to the outer layer of the cortex than is ideal. And it is often associated with toxic exposure, such as to drugs, alcohol, or environmental toxins, infection, or oxygen deprivation at some point in the past. "We have also seen it in widespread trauma," she said.

"I read that the brain perceives any traumatic event as an injury, and that you can see physical evidence of emotional injury in the brain. Is that how you could account for trauma having the same impact to the brain as a head trauma?"

"Yes. Trauma is an emotional response to an event that a person finds highly distressing. The event can be emotional or physical. The brain doesn't know the difference, only that it experienced something that caused psychological stress."

I leaned forward. "The primary difference between the person who experiences tragedy but does not have a trauma response and the one who does comes down to resilience?"

"Resilience and perspective, yes," she said.

I have long thought of resilience as a kind of emotional alchemy, a soul-refining process that takes the rough, raw materials of our lives, and renders them into something valuable. A willingness to release versions of ourselves that we created to survive. And as we become more resilient, it shape-shifts, taking on different forms depending on what the moment requires. Sometimes it's the firm determination of a rock; other times it's the fluid adaptability of water. Waves crash against the shore, relentlessly, never giving up. With each crash, they shape the shoreline, carving out new paths.

"Let's look at another set of scans, which will show the second reason I said there was likely childhood trauma. Look here." She pointed to the red areas on the scan. "You have a very active resting brain. When we compare it to the average non-traumatized brain of healthy women thirty-eight to fifty, healthy meaning without a psychiatric diagnosis, there are four areas where you have significantly increased blood flow activity. These four areas together—the thalamus, the basal ganglia, and the anterior cingulate gyrus—form this red diamond-shaped pattern right here, which is very typical in people who have survived trauma. This activation is the brain asking, 'Is the world a safe place?'"

"I know the answer is yes," I told Dr. Brush, my voice catching with emotion. "I know that the world is a safe place. But it seems as though my brain, it's slow to receive the message. Is this a manifestation of anxiety?" I shifted in my chair and quickly added, "I have never considered myself an anxious person."

"If I didn't have your history and your total brain assessment, and I just looked at your brain scans, I would have predicted debilitating depression and anxiety," she said in earnest. The truth sat heavy in my chest. Her words were humbling.

"You're an excellent example of taking what looks like a traumatized brain and making the absolute best of it. At lower levels, activation of the thalamus and basal ganglia can actually help with inner motivation. And from what I know about you, you have a lot of inner motivation." Her words were a bittersweet blend of admiration and compassion. She continued, "Some of the most highly motivated individuals we've scanned—entrepreneurs, corporate CEOs—also have significantly increased activity in this part of the brain. I would suggest your innate intelligence and self-reflection, your inner motivation, your ability to be positive, and your ability to envision—that cognitive flexibility—have really served you well."

I had turned my wounds into some kind of wisdom.

18

POST-TRAUMATIC

The next morning, I found myself drawn to connect with Grandma in the only way that felt right—through meditation. I set my intention, cued up a twenty-minute sound bath, and prepared myself. Sitting on one of my dining chairs, feet firmly on the floor, I closed my eyes, letting my arms rest gently in my lap, palms up. I rolled my neck and shoulders, easing the tension away. My breath fell into its natural rhythm: four counts in, hold for four seconds, exhale for six.

I began the visualization, imagining myself walking into a forest. In my mind's eye, the verdant canopy overhead filtered the bright sun, casting a dappled pattern on the ground, as if the forest floor were woven with memories. As I continued along a gently worn path, bark and branches crunched underfoot. White and pink wildflowers surfaced through the forest floor, signaling spring. I walked until I reached the heart of the forest and stopped in a clearing of sunlight, standing in a protective circle of light.

The silence deepened. The image flickered at first, distant and elusive, but with each breath, it gained clarity, and I felt her presence enveloping me. I could only envision her as I had known her as a child, her hair in large fluffy curls styled away from her face, above round, plastic oversized eyeglasses that came to a slight soft point just above her eyebrows. The frames were in a soft transparent brown that matched the color of her hair. She smiled. We stood facing each other in the flecked light, our eyes locking in a gaze that transcended time and space. Thirty-four years. I felt the ache of loss pulsing in me like a heartbeat in my stomach. I conveyed my love and longing to her. There were no words. In this meditative realm, we did not speak; the exchange between us was one of psychic understanding. The forest around us seemed to pulse with life, as if attuned to the rhythms of our communion, and Grandma emanated an aura of calm reassurance, as if to say that the roots of our connection could never be severed.

The circle gently fell away, and I allowed myself to come back to the present, back to my body, back into my house. With my conscious and subconscious mind working in tandem, I immediately began to free write in my journal, bringing forth whatever wanted to surface. I began:

You came to me in the forest. I have been trying to summon you in my dreams, but you did not come. I haven't seen you in so long. You had to leave. I know. I think you somehow knew it was time. But I needed you. And now, I struggle to remember you. I struggle to remember us together. I can't picture your hands. I no longer know what you smell like. Thank you for forgiving me for forgetting.

My hand didn't stop, but suddenly, she was responding.

You don't have to remember every detail. I'm with you. I am part of you. When I left, I left part of me in you. The part that feels able to do anything. The part of you that is the rebel, the thoughtful rule-breaker that does things on your own terms. That's you as well. I'm here to make sure you are always in touch with it. But you don't have to remember every detail. We didn't get much time together, not enough for you to make many memories. But I remember. I haven't missed a day since you were born. You had a lot to forget. I understand how I could get lost in that. When we try to block out the darkness, we also block out the light. You will always have questions. You would even if I was still there.

We are not promised certain outcomes, only the endless pursuit. The deliberate, curious life is not about having all the answers, but about daring to ask the questions that shape our becoming. And then living them. Embracing the gaps, the voids—they are where your sadness is meant to settle. Making space for the sorrow and the emptiness. On the other side is a transformation forged in the fires of what we cannot change.

A cherished memory, among the very few that emerge effortlessly, came to me. It paints a scene of us nestled in Grandma's backyard, where she is immersed in the ritual of her garden. Even in the warmth of summer, she would be in jeans (reserved for this particular kind of chore) paired with a slightly oversized button-down shirt. Kneeling with grace over orderly rows of soil, she introduced life into the earth, planting zucchini, squash, and mustard and collard greens.

In this sacred act, she allowed me to assist, my hands cradled in hers to steady the gardening trowel, my strength guided to loosen the soil. I became the steward of the seeds, reading aloud a packet's instructions and committing the plant's care to memory until the cartons were discarded. Before offering me the seeds, Grandma would hold them in her cupped hand, a quiet prayer, an intention for how they would grow in the world, that they would receive nourishment so that they would nourish us.

I see how perhaps she gave me everything I needed in our short time together: a love of the earth, an unwavering commitment to growth, the wisdom of nurturing life.

I began to contemplate the nature of post-traumatic growth—the silent strength that comes not from what happens to us, but from how we choose to respond. Once upon a time, I would have mistakenly believed that being post-traumatic signaled an end to the ordeal, that somehow, I had crossed an invisible threshold and could claim a medal as a participant on the other side. But what happens after is only the beginning. On the other side of loss, of trauma, of fear is where we find the invitation to become who we have the capacity to become. What we choose to do next is the pivotal crossroads of reinvention.

The post-traumatic is not a destination; it's a continual becoming, a relentless evolution.

How did I become this?

I chose to find strength in the broken places. I chose to leave behind the familiar pain of the past, to enter therapy, to confront the demons that danced in memory's dark corners, to believe the world is a safe place. I hadn't made these decisions with much fanfare; they were made with a quiet resolve that resonated through my core. As I got older, I was propelled by the belief that my life was not meant to be an anthology of suffering. My strength didn't reside just in healed wounds; it lived in the very act of survival.

There had been a time when I showed signs of PTSD. But I had shown much more than that. I had summoned the will to pick up the fragments, to examine each jagged edge, and to carefully, lovingly, decide how they fit into the narrative of who I was becoming. I found beauty in the reassembly. This is another kind of post-traumatic—the one that leads to growth. Tender green shoots of possibility pushed through the cracks of despair. The things that could have broken me didn't. I had chosen to use my trauma as a compass, pointing me toward the possibility of something more, something mine. I am made of all that I choose. My identity wasn't formed by what happened to me, but by who I decided to become.

This alternate road to healing lays bare a profound truth that shatters the confines of conventional understanding— the awakening of a spirit that defies the paradigm of perpetual suffering that in psychology has come to be known as post-traumatic growth (PTG). A theory as profound as it is perplexing, suggesting that out of the darkest moments of our lives, we can emerge not just intact, but stronger and more resilient than before. In the mid-1990s psychologists Richard Tedeschi, PhD, and Lawrence Calhoun, PhD, chose to explore the aftermath of trauma in a different light. Their encounters with veterans, widows, and survivors revealed narratives that contradicted commonly held beliefs about trauma. They observed individuals who, despite enduring unspeakable tragedy, and grappling with profound grief and pain, arose with a newfound sense of strength and purpose.

From these encounters, they determined that people diagnosed with PTSD could also be positively transformed by trauma, manifesting in five distinct phases: greater personal strength, awareness of new possibilities, strengthened relationships, an enhanced appreciation for life, and spiritual growth. While not everyone may experience all five phases of PTG, many encounter more than one. Driven by these transformations, Tedeschi and Calhoun coined the term "post-traumatic growth" to capture the essence of this phenomenon. PTG shattered the prevailing belief that traumatic experiences only leave lasting damage.

Drawn to the resonance of my own experience in this theory, I delved into further research on PTG to understand the catalytic events that inspire it. A second study from Tedeschi and Calhoun reported that social support emerges as a consistent predictor of growth; individuals who perceive greater support from family, friends, and communities are more likely to experience PTG. Additionally, coping strategies such as meaning making are associated with higher levels of growth, suggesting that how individuals process and make sense of their experiences influences their ability to grow in the aftermath of trauma.

I began tracing the contours of my own story with a newfound sense of clarity. I understood the power of community. I had many friends that felt like family—incredible women who had shown me the protective and nurturing strength of sisterhood and men who helped me understand my own. In their presence, I was both anchored and set free, seen without feeling exposed, learning that sometimes the deepest spiritual answers are found in human connections that science cannot measure. In the embrace of these relationships, I experienced some of my most profound healing, and I saw my own capacity for love, compassion, and connection expand.

More than finding meaning, Tedeschi and Calhoun found *benefits* of the experience.

I couldn't stop reading.

In 2006, researchers Vicki S. Helgeson, Kerry A. Reynolds, and Patricia L. Tomich delved into the relationship between benefit finding and psychological health through a meta-analysis on PTG. Their findings, published in the *Journal of Consulting and Clinical Psychology*, highlighted that benefit finding was associated with less depression and a greater sense of well-being, although it also entailed more intrusive and avoidant thoughts about the stressor. Many psychologists refer to these constructs as a form of cognitive processing, attempts to understand traumatic events, rather than markers of mental health.

> Some might argue that a period of contemplation and consideration of the stressor is necessary for growth to occur. To the extent that intrusive and avoidant thoughts are markers of cognitive processing rather than of distress, the relation of benefit finding to these thoughts makes more sense and is not necessarily inconsistent with relations of benefit finding to reduced depression and greater positive affect.

This growth, they found, is often more pronounced in women, in people of non-white heritage, and in individuals from modest means—all populations that have been tempered by adversity and shaped by the collective wisdom of generations. From the wisdom of age to the fortitude of womanhood, from the communal bonds of collectivist cultures and the spirit of those from impoverished backgrounds, the demographic findings painted a portrait of resilience in all its diverse manifestations. They painted a portrait of my story, a purposeful reconstruction, a deliberate act of creating something sacred from the profane. Of finding the good in the bad, of laughing to keep from crying, as the saying goes.

And there it was—the truth of cognitive restructuring, the alchemy of turning pain into power. Each negative experience, once a source of anguish, became a stepping stone toward understanding and strength. Trauma changes the brain. So does healing.

Every day for a year, those burlap-covered mounds stood to highlight the fickleness of expectation. Each glance out my front window served as a stark reminder that we will always face things beyond our control. The burlap, once a symbol of defeat, gradually took on a new meaning, a reminder that even when beauty is veiled, it remains, gathering strength in the unseen places.

It was time to move them. I knelt beside the first bush and removed the burlap, a quiet prayer. There among the dry, chewed-up spindly branches were small bright green leaves. Its roots, unseen yet vital, snaked beneath the surface, grasping for life in the sandy soil. I dug my fingers into the earth as I carefully worked around the base of the bush.

The roots resisted at first, clinging to the familiarity of their surroundings. The push-pull of leaving behind the world they'd come to know, even if it was one that wouldn't be good for them. But with gentle insistence, I persisted, easing the plant from its cradle and carrying it from the front of the house to the back and up the stairs to the deck.

"First one down," I announced triumphantly, holding the bush in my arms like a newborn. Its roots dangled, vulnerable and exposed. With great care, I nestled the first hydrangea into its planter. The rich soil welcomed the plant with a promise, one that affirmed protection and new beginnings. I pressed the earth around its base. "I hope you will thrive here."

I moved to the next, then the next, finding a rhythm in the steady work. For two full days, I dug them up, cleaned their roots, trimmed away the old, and placed them in fresh dirt. By the time the twelfth bush was nestled alongside the others, my body ached for rest, but my spirit was lighter than it had been in years. One by one, the hydrangeas took to their new homes, the sparse little leaves reaching toward the sun with what seemed like gratitude. Standing back, I surveyed the row of planters, a mother taking pride in her children. They were still small, still struggling, but mine. With each bit of water I poured into their soil, I poured in my hope, too, as if they could understand my fervent desire for their survival. The front garden, now dotted with empty spaces, didn't look like defeat. It looked like possibility. An opportunity for something new that could flourish there.

The days melted into each other, each morning unwrapping itself with the tender promise of a fresh start. I tended to my hydrangeas with the kind of focused attention I had once reserved for the more elusive ambitions of my life. That first summer of nurturing passed with the slowness of honey dripping from a spoon. Each day I watched and waited, knowing that the true measure of growth was not always visible to the naked eye. Even when there were no signs of progress, I kept watering, kept nurturing, kept believing in the potential of what was yet unseen.

The second summer arrived with a quiet sense of hope. The bare stems of last year had thickened, those skeletal remains had given way to something that bore the markings of life.

"Look at you," I gasped, a smile tugging at the corners of my mouth as I spoke to them like old friends. "You made it. We did it."

They stood there, lush and quiet, their fullness a far cry from the brittle beginnings of the year before. And there, amid the green, the first white blooms unfurled, delicate and resilient. Proof that life could return, even after what felt like a devastating ending.

We carry that same power in us—to rise again, to transform, to flourish against all odds. To stretch toward the light, even after being buried. We can still grow. Still, we become. And in those quiet moments, when new life finally breaks through, we remember that we were always meant to be.

ACKNOWLEDGMENTS

In *The Dictionary of Obscure Sorrows,* John Koenig gives voice to the inexpressible nature of the human condition through a lexicon of brilliant, newly minted words. Among them, one resonates with a particular poignancy at this very moment: *suerza.* It's a combination of the Spanish words *suerte,* meaning luck, and *fuerza,* meaning force. And luck-force is exactly what this moment feels like, or some combination of the two. But *suerza* is defined as a feeling of quiet amazement that you exist at all; a sense of gratitude that you were even born in the first place, that you somehow emerged alive and breathing despite all odds, having won an unbroken streak of reproductive lotteries that stretches all the way back to the beginning of life itself.

All of my love to those who have taken on the role of family, offering a safe place for me to be and become. There are too many of you to name, another reminder of my extraordinary fortune. You allowed me to disappear to write this book while checking in on me—calling, voice noting, inviting me even when I'd say, "Not this time," and keeping me tethered when my solitude threatened to pull me deeper into myself. Thank you for not letting me drown. I love you.

To my darling Nikki (Tamu Nicole Brooks, because I want your full name in print), thank you for being my favorite cousin and family historian. I am grateful for your guidance, for allowing me to call upon your memory, and for your unwavering love and support. You have always cheered me on; please know I'm rooting for you, too.

To Dr. and Mrs. Ivery, you showed me love, grace, and acceptance at a time when I needed it most. I've never been able to truly thank you for your kindness and generosity. Please know that it has always meant so much to me, perhaps more now than ever.

To Eric Nargi, thank you for taking care of my home (and therefore, my sanity). You had a front-row seat to months of my writing process. I appreciate the kindness and compassion you showed me during that time.

Deep gratitude to my friends and early readers—Tracey Bey Johnson, Myron Branford, and Maxie McCoy—thank you for your time, your brilliance, your insight and feedback, your kind words, and your great care. I'm honored.

To Emily Sweet, this book's true Day One, I am so grateful for your encouragement of me telling this story a decade before I was ready, and for being my obvious choice when I knew it was time. I am forever in your debt. You are the reason I am part of the Park & Fine Literary and Media family.

Which brings me to my agents, Mia Vitale and Sarah Passick: Thank you for your belief in this project, for getting it an audience with some of the best in the business, and for your support of my debut throughout the process.

Jessica Sindler, this book wouldn't be what it is without you. You are my friend and my literary soul sister. I am in awe of your intelligence and your instincts and have profound gratitude for your wise and sympathetic counsel, always offering the perfect balance of reassurance and perspective. I love you, lady.

To my publisher, Krishan Trotman, thank you for seeing and supporting my vision, for loving my writing, for pushing me to dig deep, and for bringing the storyteller out of me and onto the page. Thank you to the rest of the talented Legacy Lit team—Amina, Maya, Leah, and Mahito—and the greater Hachette Book Group organization for your hard work in bringing this book to the world.

With gratitude,
Daria

12 301